M000116839

THRIVING

— IN THE —
SECOND HALF OF LIFE

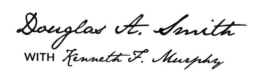

Douglas A. Smith
WITH Kenneth F. Murphy

Published by
White Pine Mountain
445 Hutchinson Ave., Ste 270
Columbus, OH 43235

Copyright © 2020 by Douglas A. Smith
& Kenneth F. Murphy

Edited by RobinLee Allen

Cover design and layout by
Summerfield Advertising

Illustrations by
Michael West

ISBN: 978-0-9860708-3-9

Library of Congress Control Number: 2020941806

All Rights Reserved. No parts of this book may be
reproduced or transmitted in any form or by any means,
electronic or mechanical, including photocopying,
recording, or by any information storage and retrieval
system without written permission from the author,
except for the inclusion of brief quotations in a review.

Printed in the United States of America.

"The Child is father to the man."
—William Wordsworth

For Gordon and Greg

Your mother and I could not have two finer sons.
You have shaped our lives in so many wonderful
ways. May your lives be filled with joy and love …
may you both thrive.

Love,

Dad

TABLE OF CONTENTS

PREFACE

On the evening of Sept. 1, 2004, I was sitting in a hematologist office at the Mayo Clinic after two full days of testing to determine the cause of a somewhat strange MRI I'd had a month earlier back in Columbus, Ohio. After numerous tests, they could seem to find nothing wrong. As I was about to leave Dr. White's office with what seemed like a clean bill of health, just like in the movies, the phone rings. The doctor listens intently, hangs up, jots down a few notes, then slowly turns to me and in a soft, compassionate voice tells me that based on the pathology report, I have an incurable form of blood cancer.*

In almost all great literature there is an "inciting incident." Some major, unexpected, unwelcomed event occurs that forces the protagonist to reconsider the fabric of his or her life. I didn't realize it then, but Dr. White's unexpected diagnosis was my inciting incident and the launching point of the second half of my life.

On that day at the Mayo Clinic, my life changed. Change often happens in an instant. A life-changing diagnosis, an accident, the loss of a loved one ... these changes can happen in seconds. What does not happen in an instant, as I have painfully discovered, is the transition required to deal with the change. Major transitions take time, often years, and involve what James Hollis calls traveling through the "neutral zone," or what he even more accurately describes as the "swampland." The journey through the swampland is almost never without pain and a deep sense of loss and confusion, but the swampland also offers us the opportunity for new perspectives, new insights, in fact new life, if we are persistent and open to what the swampland has to offer.

With my inciting incident, like most protagonists, I resisted entering the swampland. First by ignoring its calling altogether and then seeking to simply escape by quitting my work. I found a blank calendar was not a blessing, but an incredible curse as I experienced a deep and enduring depression — not an uncommon state of mind for those entering the swampland. Over a year later, with the help of my loving wife and excellent professional care, I began to emerge from my depression. Emerging from the depression did not end the swampland, but it did open me to the messages its pain and confusion had to offer. I found the swampland is indeed a dismal place, but one filled with opportunity for new growth, new perspectives and the development of a deeper more resilient self. Without the swampland, I would have remained driven by the needs and desires of the first half of life and I would have failed to enter into the richness offered by the second half.

I think for most of us, the first half of life has to fall apart before we move to the depth and clarity of the second half. As long as the way we carry forth in the first half seems to be working, there is little incentive to change what we do or how we think. What's more, the invitation to the second half is often not very attractive. Mine certainly wasn't. The reality is that most people will have an inciting incident that pushes them toward the second half of life and forces, or at least suggests, the need to re-evaluate. The incident will be different for everyone. Job loss, divorce, illness, the death of a loved one, our changing physical abilities as we age, or some combination of several of these tend to be most common. Some will reject this invitation to the second half. This book is written for those who don't.

Although moving into the second half of life was not easy, I have found it to be an incredibly beautiful journey. In the 16 years since Dr. White's diagnosis launched me into the second half, my life has been richer, deeper and more meaningful. How I think, what I do, how I interact with others, my attitude, my gratitude, how I invest my humble talents — all of it, I believe, better serves me, my family and the world. I have come to love this stage of my life. I have evolved from being driven to being inspired, from pleasing my ego to honoring my conscience, from accumulating wealth to contributing wealth, from worrying about status to longing for significance, from doing what others expect of me to honoring what my soul is aching for. I love the view from the second half of life.

I have come to believe that to live a full life, to thrive, or as the science of positive psychology puts it, to "flourish," the second half has to be different from the first, and I am afraid the only way to make this journey to the second half is through the swampland. This book is intended to help guide people on this journey.

In 2014 I wrote "Happiness: The Art of Living with Peace, Confidence and Joy." The book focused on 13 skills that I believe lead to peace about the past, confidence in the future and joy in the present. Much of what I shared was based on the emerging science of positive psychology. In the intervening six years, I have come to better understand the science of positive psychology and these 13 skills. I have also come to see them in the context of the second half of life. In this book, with the help of my friend Ken Murphy, I have tried to deepen the reader's understanding of these same skills and to see them through the lens of life's second half. Readers of my previous book will find considerable overlap. My hope is that the repetition, coupled with new insights and new tools, will enrich your understanding of the 13 skills and help you better practice them in the second half of life.

The book is structured to illuminate the skills that can lead to thriving in the second half of life and to encourage personal reflection. After an overview of positive psychology, which is the foundation of the 13 skills, Ken shares the intimate details that pushed him into the second half of his life. Then in the following chapters, I dive into the individual skills that lead to peace with the past and confidence in the future, how to live with greater resilience, the skills that lead to finding joy in the present, and finally the dead ends many of us head down in our search for happiness. The final chapter reveals an additional skill that underlies all 13 skills.

At the end of each chapter, Ken and I included questions for reflection and quotes related to what is covered in the chapter. We wanted to share the many thought-provoking ideas others have had about the second half of life with the goal of inspiring your own epiphanies.

I never anticipated the diagnosis I received on Sept. 1,

2004, could lead to a second half of life so full of peace and happiness. I hope you find this book both enjoyable and helpful in your own search for a second half of life full of joy, meaning and accomplishment. I hope you thrive.

— Douglas A. Smith

*When I was diagnosed in 2004 there were no treatments for my blood cancer that extended life. My life expectancy was roughly five to 10 years. As I write this today, over 16 years later, I am taking part in a trial of ACP-196, an experimental medicine. Most of my blood counts are now close to normal and if this drug has a side-effect, I don't know what it is. On November 19, 2019, ACP-196 was approved by the FDA and is now available to all who suffer from my illness under the brand name Acalabrutinib. I am deeply indebted to the doctors, researchers and pharmaceutical companies that discover and develop these drugs. I am particularly grateful to Ahmed Hamdy, Raquel Izumi and Tasheda Navarro, who originally developed this drug, and to the James Cancer Center, Dr. John Byrd and his team who managed its trial and secured its approval. I would not be here if it were not for these people. Thank you.

Chapter 1

POSITIVE PSYCHOLOGY & EMOTIONS

Flourishing is living within an optimal range of human functioning, one that connotes goodness, generativity, growth and resilience.
—BARBARA FREDRICKSON & MARCIAL LOSADA

Flourishing

In the years after my diagnosis, the question of what led to a joyful, meaningful life consumed many of my waking hours. The full realization that my time on this earth was limited — and out of my control — had a way of focusing my attention. If I had some 2,000 to 3,000 days left, I suppose I wanted to use them most effectively.

We don't have to guess anymore what leads to a joyful, meaningful, accomplished life, what the science of positive psychology refers to as "flourishing." To capture it most succinctly, flourishing is the experience of life going well. Flourishing is both feeling good and functioning effectively — it epitomizes good mental health. Since the advent of positive psychology, there has been an explosion in the amount of research concerning the topic of happiness. Science may now back up much of what your grandparents probably told you about living a happy life, and, importantly, the science adds significant new insights.

The science of positive psychology emerged in 1998 when Martin Seligman, then head of the American Psychological Association, proposed that psychology could play a bigger role in helping people than it was at that time. He pointed out that the science of psychology was devoted almost entirely to the 20% of the population with some form of pathological issue. While this focus resulted in many advances that helped those suffering from numerous forms of mental illness, he felt psychologists could help the other 80% as well by helping all people live more joyful, meaningful and accomplished lives. At first, positive psychologists worked with the goal of helping more people achieve lasting happiness. However, they saw "happiness" as something far deeper than merely pleasure or hedonics. In fact, they outlined three separate routes to happiness, as well as a fourth route that was a combination of the first three.

Routes to Happiness

1. Pleasure: The idea here is to have life be one glorious vacation, a life devoted to maximizing positive emotions. One does this by planning to do more pleasant activities. If you like hiking, do more of it. If you like having dinner with friends, schedule it regularly. The problem with this route is that a life devoted to pleasure is the least effective route to happiness. Pleasure is unavoidably fleeting, so it becomes difficult to sustain a life based on pleasure. Additionally, at some point, most of us begin to wonder, "What is my life all about? What is the meaning of all this?" This route offers no answer to this burning question.

2. Engagement: A second route to happiness is pursuing activities that use our strengths, our skills. Most of us have spent a good deal of our lives doing this. We figure out what our strengths are and then engage in activities that make the most of them at work and play. Developing our strengths and using them provides a more sustainable and deeper level of satisfaction than pleasure alone. But it still leaves a question around meaning. As Seligman points out, he is skilled at duplicate bridge and he enjoys competing, but if he spends too much time playing duplicate bridge, he begins to wonder if he is wasting his life. Using our strengths to do things we enjoy is a great route to happiness, but for most of us, it isn't enough. It takes a third route to achieve true happiness.

3. Meaning: The third route to happiness is engagement plus. It is not only using our strengths but using them in service to others. Meaning is the route that brings the greatest long-term gratification of the three routes. It raises our self-esteem, our sense of purpose and our sense of well-being. Interestingly, neither engagement nor meaning produce as immediate a result as pleasure. In fact, these routes can bring discomfort or occasional feelings of stress and anxiety. They can even dampen short-term pleasantness. Watching your 10-year-old daughter play a baseball game on a cold rainy day or relentlessly training for a marathon may not be pleasurable, but both of these activities can lead to gratification and happiness.

4. The Full Life: The full life is having the ability to use all three routes to happiness: to experience positive emotions and pleasure, to know and use our strengths and to be in service to the larger community. People who use all three routes take the time to savor life's pleasures, they know themselves well enough to know what they do well and use these strengths in their everyday life, and they find something meaningful to which to devote their time and effort. The full life leads to a life of meaning, fulfillment and joy ... it leads to the ability to flourish.

Source: "A Balanced Psychology and a Full Life," Seligman, Parks & Steen, The Royal Society, August 2004

As positive psychologists were mapping out the four routes to happiness, they were also identifying the role of various factors in determining our happiness.

While heredity and circumstances play a role in our happiness, positive psychology was founded on the belief that we could increase our happiness — that happiness was a skill to be developed. From their work emerged a formula that suggested happiness was the result of a set point (heredity) plus circumstances and voluntary choices (skill).

$$H = S + C + V$$

HAPPINESS = Set Point + Circumstances + Voluntary Choices

Through their research, positive psychologists discovered that about 50% of our happiness was determined by our biological parents; about 10% was due to circumstances; and about 40% was determined by voluntary choices, or how we choose to perceive and respond to our circumstances. I think the number that is most surprising in their analysis is that circumstances account for only about 10% of how happy we are. In the short term, a major setback or positive life change (a severe accident or winning the lottery) can have a major impact on our happiness. But in the longer term (six months to a year), we most likely will return to the happiness level we experienced before the event.

Since we can't do a damn thing about our heredity (except pick good parents), we won't spend time on this aspect of happiness. Instead, we'll focus on the 50% of our happiness we can influence. Through our voluntary choices, we can clearly affect our circumstances and recent research even shows these choices can raise our set point.

Most positive psychologists eventually gave up on "happiness" as the word to capture the core of their work, as it was just too difficult to change people's perspective on what it means to be happy. Instead, they began to focus on enabling humans across the globe to "flourish." There are several definitions of flourishing, but perhaps the positive psychologist Barbara Fredrickson captures it most effectively as: "Flourishing is living within an optimal range of human functioning, one that connotes goodness, generativity, growth and resilience."

Throughout this book, I have used "to be happy," "to

flourish," and "to thrive" interchangeably, with a belief that each of these is consistent with this definition.

People who flourish have a set of attributes that is perhaps most easily, if not completely, captured by the letters **PERMASOR**, an acronym for:

1. Positive Emotions: They experience many more positive emotions (e.g., joy, gratitude, serenity, hope, pride, interest, awe, love) and fewer negative emotions (e.g., anger, jealousy, envy, hopelessness, shame). They do this both subliminally and consciously. All things considered they are happier.

2. Engagement: They are engaged in life. They are interested and interesting. They love to learn new things and are open to new experiences.

3. Relationships: They have enduring and healthy relationships. They find that there are people in their life that deeply care about them and this care is returned.

4. Meaning: They believe that their life has meaning, purpose and value. They use their talents to make a difference in the world.

5. Accomplishment: They are clear about what they wish to achieve in life and set goals, the achievement of which gives them a sense of accomplishment.

6. Self-Esteem: They feel both confident and worthy. They are confident they can face the challenges life throws their way and they feel worthy of happiness, recognizing that they, like all of us, will make mistakes from which they can recover, learn and move on.

7. Optimism: They feel positively about the future. They don't expend energy contemplating unnecessary "what ifs" and "if onlys." When negative events occur, they perceive them as temporary, limited in scope (they don't catastrophize) and, if not controllable, they believe they can at least act to influence the outcome. They accept the mystery of life.

8. Resilience: When they experience setbacks, they bounce back quickly because they have each of the prior seven attributes. They are immune to "learned helplessness" and they often experience "post-traumatic growth" (PTG), learning and growing from these experiences.

The 13 skills presented in this book, when consistently practiced, enable us to possess the attributes of PERMASOR; they enable us to flourish.

Countries ranked by percent of population flourishing

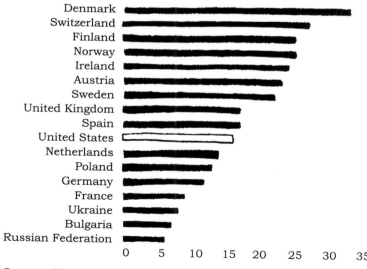

Source: Flourish: A Visionary New Understanding of Happiness and Well-being," Martin Seligman, U.S. statistic added separately

So in which countries are people flourishing? To answer this question, two researchers at University of Cambridge set out to survey residents in 23 different countries. With over 2,000 respondents from each country, here are the results: Denmark is highest, with a score of 33%. The Russian Federation is lowest, with a score of 6%. Positive psychologists estimate that in the United States only 16% of our citizens are flourishing.

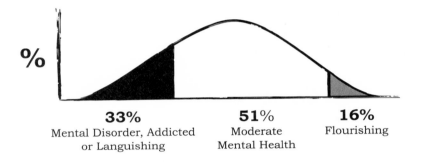

33%	**51%**	**16%**
Mental Disorder, Addicted or Languishing	Moderate Mental Health	Flourishing

Source: Oxford Handbook of Positive Psychology, Oxford University Press, 2011

While only 16% of us are flourishing, twice as many, or 33%, are languishing. Languishing is defined as suffering from some form of mental illness, addiction to alcohol or drugs, or not functioning well psychologically or socially. Positive psychologists are committed to enabling more people to flourish, moving this bell curve to the right.

Like positive psychologists, my goal with this book is to enable more of us to flourish. Imagine if we could reverse these numbers, so that 33% of people in the U.S. are flourishing and only 16% are languishing. Martin Seligman has set a goal for positive psychology to have 51% of the world's population flourishing by 2051.

There are numerous benefits to flourishing. Study after study suggests we do better, in every domain of our lives, if we flourish. (Two of the most famous of the studies documenting the benefits of living with joy are the "Nun Study" and the "Mills College Yearbook Study," both of which you can easily find online.)

Here's how Ed Diener, a leading positive psychologist, captures the benefits of flourishing. We:

- Live longer/succumb to fewer illnesses

- Have more friends/more enduring relationships

- Have better and longer marriages

- Commit fewer crimes/are less likely to hurt others

- Are more creative and expansive in our thinking

- Work harder/do better at work/make more money

- Are less likely to be addicted to alcohol/drugs

- Help others more*

*Source: "Happiness: Unlocking the Mysteries of Psychological Wealth," Ed Diener

I believe people who flourish have a unique perspective on three things:

1. They have peace with the past.

They do not carry a lot of remorse and or anger about the past. Rather they learn from their experiences and then find ways to move on, letting these negative emotions go.

2. They have confidence in the future.

They recognize they have a role in preparing for the future, but they also realize they cannot control the future. Therefore, they focus on what they can do and are prepared to accept and adjust to whatever unforeseen diversions the universe takes as the future unfolds.

3. They live in the present.

With the ability to let go of the past and have confidence in the future, people who flourish are free to live in the present with joy and exuberance.

People who flourish have a sense of ballast in their lives that enables them to go through traumas — a lost job, a broken relationship, a health challenge, or most anything life throws at them — and still eventually return to a sense of well-being and contentment. In effect, they bounce back. When such people face setbacks, they move more quickly through the Kübler-Ross "Stages of Grief " — denial, anger, bargaining, depression and acceptance. They are more resilient.

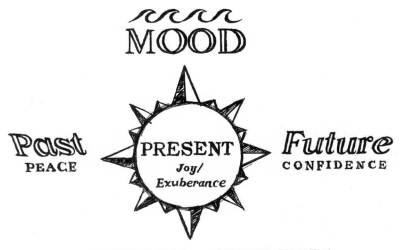

CONTENTMENT *and* WELL-BEING

I further believe that what enables people who flourish to have these perspectives is a set of 13 skills that come out of the science of positive psychology. Each of these skills plays an important role in enabling us to flourish. This book is designed to help you better understand these skills and how they lead to flourishing, as well as provide tools to better practice these skills.

Skills to Flourish

Past	Present	Future
1. Forgiveness	3. Doing Now What I'm Doing Now	10. Faith
2. Gratitude	4. Honoring Mind/Body/Spirit	11. Optimism
	5. Being Altruistic/Kind	12. Flexibility
	6. Thinking with Abundance	13. Openness
	7. Mastering Our Stories	(FOFO)
	8. Finding Meaning/Purpose	
	9. Cherishing Relationships	

These skills take on increasing importance in the second half of life. For instance, without forgiveness, we can carry an increasing burden of remorse and anger from the accumulation of hurts we have experienced or caused. The blackbird of guilt and the curse of anger can prevent us from experiencing the joy available to us in later years.

Emotions

Each of the 13 skills we will cover are deeply affected by and affect our emotions. So before we dive into the skills, let's spend some time understanding emotions — what they are, their origins, the role they play in our ability to flourish and, importantly, how to manage them better.

Emotions, both positive and negative, are short-lived experiences that determine how we feel, think and act. They therefore play a critical role in our lives. The word "emotions" comes from the Greek word "emote" or "to move." While we experience both positive and negative emotions, most of us experience far more negative emotions than positive emotions, and far more than we need to.

We experience more negative emotions in part because they are more enduring, or as positive psychologists say, they are "sticky." This is a legacy of evolution in that negative emotions are key to survival because they protect us from harm. Our emotional responses are biased toward correcting mistakes and recognizing danger, rather than reflecting on what went well. Evolution has seen to it that we remember failures more than successes and that we spend more time analyzing bad events than good ones. In a sense, we have learned to be Velcro to the negative events in our lives and Teflon to the positive events.

There is even a special hormone, norepinephrine, that our mind triggers when we perceive a significant traumatic event. Norepinephrine works to ingrain the negative event into our hippocampus, making the memory more difficult to erase.

However, emotions are not simply a result of some event; stimulus does not necessarily equal response. In truth, no one and nothing necessarily makes us feel a particular way. We have a choice in our emotional response to an event — even if that choice does not seem evident. We create our own emotions; and if we create them, we can change them. We choose our emotions — to be angry, jealous, anxious or to be happy. Managing our emotional responses is a difficult, but essential part of flourishing.

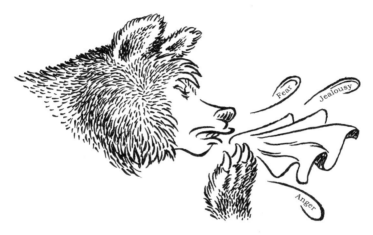

Emotions are contagious. When someone smiles, we naturally smile back. Negative emotions are particularly contagious. Negative emotions include fear, anger, disgust, sadness, jealousy, shame, derision, contempt and anxiety. When we experience these emotions, we cultivate them in those around us. Emotions signal others to either approach us or avoid us.

Negative emotions play an important role in our lives. Fear warns us that something might harm us and to avoid it; anger gets us to protect ourselves from someone who is not treating us appropriately; disgust causes us to regurgitate or avoid something that could be harmful; sadness encourages us to stop and reflect, regroup. But once these negative emotions have played their role, we often continue to hold on to them ... for years. When we hang on to anger, remorse or other negative emotions long after they have served their purpose, they become destructive. They cause us to experience what psychologists call "dirty pain." I believe these unprocessed negative emotions are often stored in the body and eventually manifest as illness.

Positive emotions also play a very important role in our lives. **Below are the 10 most common positive emotions and various actions they inspire:**

Joy — Curiosity, Energy, Play

Gratitude — Generosity, Satisfaction

Serenity — Reflection, Integration, Spirituality

Hope — Optimism, Seeking Positive Change

Interest — Pursuit of Knowledge

Pride — Self-esteem, Confidence

Amusement — Creativity, Openness

Inspiration — Desire to Excel

Awe — Openness, Gratitude, Spirituality

Love — All of the Above

The happiest among us, those people who flourish, experience more positive emotions and they do this both consciously and subconsciously. Positive emotions don't just feel good, they enable us to perform better in life and at work. As Barbara Fredrickson stated in her "Broaden and Build Theory," when we experience positive emotions, we are more open, more creative, better at problem-solving, more receptive to the thoughts and ideas of others, and we make better friends, better teammates, better leaders. Positive emotions broaden our thinking and attention, they make us more resilient and better able to deal with setbacks and crises (more on resilience later). They trigger upward spirals: Positive emotions lead to mindfulness, which leads to broadened awareness, which leads to greater connections with others and to more energy.

Negative emotions like fear, anger, disgust, do the opposite. They cause downward spirals: They narrow our focus as we ruminate about the past or have trepidation about the future, they cause us to disconnect from others, which leads to less effective relationships, which leads to less energy.

We can expand the positive emotions we feel by practicing a set of skills that make up the core of this book. We'll provide tools designed to help you practice each skill so you experience more positive emotions.

Here is a chart of both negative and positive emotions. While each of the negative emotions listed on the left side may be appropriate at certain times, to flourish we should strive to experience the positive emotions on the right side more often.

NEGATIVE EMOTIONS	POSITIVE EMOTIONS
Angry	Joyful
Resentful	Engaged
Frustrated	Loving
Defensive	Hopeful
Fearful	Amused
Anxious	Passionate
Disgusted	In the Flow
Jealous	Inspired
Cheated	Cheerful
Pressured	Awed
Intimidated	Interested
Frantic	Affectionate
Persecuted	Energetic
Ashamed	Carefree
Exhausted	Peaceful
Burned Out	Serene
Lethargic	Relieved
Defeated	Mellow
Hopeless	Relaxed
Sad	Reflective
Grieving	Grateful
Ignored	Amused
Blue	Hopeful
Helpless	Proud
Depressed	Blissful
Vulnerable	Contented
Worried	Satisfied

HIGH ENERGY (top rows), LOW ENERGY (bottom rows)

Source: Modified from material of the Human Performance Institute

Reflections for the Second Half

- Can you identify additional positive and negative emotions? (Hint: There are hundreds.)

- Where do you think you spend most of your time, on the left or right side of the chart?

- Which emotions drive or inspire your behavior?

- Which of the negative emotions do you find most "sticky"?

- How would you like to change where you spend most of your time? How might you achieve this?

Quotes About Positive Psychology/ Happiness/Flourishing

1. *"Mental Health: The successful performance of mental function, resulting in productive activities, fulfilling relationships with other people and the ability to adapt to change and to cope with adversity."*
                    —SURGEON GENERAL'S CRITERIA, 1999

2. *"I use the term happiness to refer to the experience of joy, contentment, or positive well-being, combined with a sense that one's life is good, meaningful and worthwhile."*
                    —SONJA LYUBOMIRSKY

3. *"Happiness does not come automatically. It is not a gift that good fortune bestows upon us and a reversal of fortune takes back. It depends on us alone. In order to become happy, we have to learn how to change ourselves."*
— LUIGI LUCA AND FRANCESCO CAVALLI-SFORZA

4. *"Happiness is a state of mind ... even when the surface waters churn, the deep currents run sure."*
                    —DAVID MYERS

5. *"Happiness is a state of inner fulfillment, not the gratification of inexhaustible desires for outward things."*

—MATTHIEU RICARD

6. *"Positive psychology is founded on the belief that people want to live meaningful and fulfilling lives, to cultivate what is best in themselves and to enhance their experiences of love, work and play."*

—MARTIN SELIGMAN

7. *"Happiness is the meaning and the purpose of life, the whole aim and end of human existence."*

—ARISTOTLE

8. *"How to gain, how to keep, how to recover happiness is in fact for most men at all times the secret motive of all they do, and of all they are willing to endure."*

—WILLIAM JAMES

9. *"We obtained cheerfulness data on students entering college in 1976 and then checked their income in the 1990s. The happiest quartile had an average salary that was 30% higher than the lowest quartile."*

—ED DIENER

10. *"It pays to be happy."*
                                —DOUGLAS A. SMITH

11. *"Flourishing is living within an optimal range of human functioning, one that connotes goodness, generativity, growth and resilience."*
                                —BARBARA FREDRICKSON

12. *"Happiness is having a large, loving, caring, close-knit family ... in another city."*
                                —GEORGE BURNS

13. *"The benefits of happiness include higher income and superior work outcomes (e.g., greater productivity and higher quality of work); larger social rewards (e.g., more satisfying and longer marriages, more friends, stronger social support, and richer social interactions); more activity, energy, and flow; better physical health (e.g., a bolstered immune system, lowered stress levels and less pain); and even longer life. The literature, my colleagues and I have found, also suggests that happy individuals are more creative, helpful, charitable and self-confident; have better self-control; and show great self-regulatory and coping abilities."*
                                —SONJA LYUBOMIRSKY

14. *"Flourishing elicits many tangible outcomes — self-efficacy, likability, pro-social behavior, active involvement with goal pursuit, we are more approachable, have higher motivation, greater resilience, perform better in the workplace which in turn creates positive emotions, creating an upward spiral."*

—BARBARA FREDRICKSON

Chapter 2

FINDING NEW LIFE IN OUR SECOND HALF

BY KEN MURPHY

*And then the knowledge comes to me that I have
space within me for a second, timeless, larger life.*
—RAINER MARIA RILKE

The First Half of Life

In our teens and twenties, the dominant issue we deal
with is: What does the world expect of me? According
to James Hollis, Ph.D., a Jungian psychoanalyst, it is
through this lens of others' expectations that we establish
our sense of values, place, worth, and accomplishment.

As we grow and make important choices from childhood
on — about friends, school, fields of interest, politics,
careers — outside forces heavily shape how we perceive
the world and our place in it. From the time we are born,
the experiences and views of parents, peers, teachers
and the communities we are born into influence what
we want and how we think.

Brick by brick, year by year, we build a persona — our face to the world.

We also mold our dreams in line with that emerging visage — and form a picture about what a "good" life looks like. Where do we get this image? What is it within us that informs what we supposedly want? Our parents represent an outsized influence. What they chose, along with their struggles, triumphs and disappointments, loom large in our developing sense of self. Within the example of their lives, we often see what it is we end up running toward — or away from.

My own life is an example. My father returned from the Pacific after World War II, married his college sweetheart, got a law degree, joined the first of several big companies he would work for and started on a 40-year corporate journey with many highs and lows. At 49, he built his dream house on a beach in Long Island. In his fifties, he battled to hold his senior position, weathering eight younger bosses in nine years. He had been retired just four months when his life ended, cut short by cancer. At the time of his passing at 65, he was planning the construction of a small tower of glass atop his 1970s beach house in order to take in a 360-degree view of the sound and the bay.

The third of four sons, I went to college to study labor relations. Check that — in truth, I first went to school intending to pursue television and radio. Finding my introverted self plunked into a mob of raging extroverts sent me searching for calmer ground. I drifted through economics and into labor relations. I found the dramatic and often violent history of the labor movement interesting enough, and the die was cast.

After graduation, I joined the first of several big companies I would work for, married my high school sweetheart, and started on a 30-year corporate journey, filled with highs and lows. At 48, I built my dream house on the beach — one mile from my father's house. As we started construction, I added a little something to the plan (and budget) — a small tower of glass that would take in a 360-degree view of the sound and the bay. At 50, a bad job situation, along with a stage 2 colon cancer diagnosis, triggered a major transition — and an abrupt end to my pursuit of all things corporate. It yanked me off the track that my father had taken years before ... all the way to his end. In our respective periods of midlife, our paths diverged.

In our first half, we focus primarily on becoming a responsible and productive adult, taking our rightful place in society — whatever we perceive that to be. There is nothing wrong with this — the manufactured persona we build is a necessary step we take to prove to others and to ourselves that we can indeed survive on our own in the world. Development of a strong, sturdy ego is the goal of the first half of life — and rightfully so. It is difficult to grow beyond our ego if it remains immature and unformed. But if we are to flourish in the second half of life, ego, strength and satisfaction cannot be the end of the story.

Along the way to building what Hollis calls this "provisional personality," and Richard Rohr refers to as the "false self," we often put away the so-called "childish things" — interests that once held fascination for our developing selves. Some passions indeed may have been right for their time and no more. In others, whatever they may be — service, music, art, sport, performing — we may uncover signals that may help us write the next chapter. First, children must be raised, the bills must be paid, promotions earned, an image constructed — those demands are often the main story of the first half. Quiet stirrings of what might be more central to our being are shushed in the rush to get done the task at hand. Maybe someday, we say, but not now. But the soul has its own timetable, and rarely stays quiet for long.

**Growing Gap Between Life As Constructed...
and Who We Were Meant To Be**

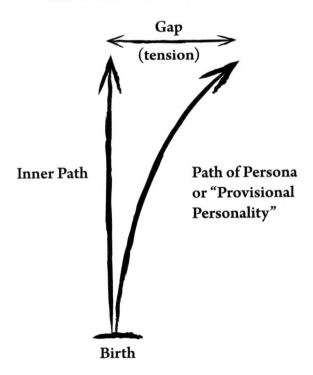

Source: James Hollis

As the gap grows between the face we put out to the world and the deepest sense of who we are at our core, the psyche finds a way to register its protest.

According to Hollis, common methods of quieting this inner voice are denial, distraction, frenzied activity ("I am soooo busy"), addiction to any number of negative options, or projecting our pain onto others. Often, our own body will powerfully signal when our way of living might be out of sync with who we really are.

At 40, even while I was moving up the corporate ladder, I was frequently seized by crippling back pain. In the middle of meetings, I would be forced to hit the floor in agony, knees hugged to chest, tossing out commentary from the prone position. Nothing helped for long — chiropractic treatment, acupuncture, stretching, even surgery. That is until I met with Dr. John Sarno, legendary for his unique treatment of back pain.

Sarno told me that in all likelihood my pain, while genuine, was not caused by a physical abnormality but rather by emotional tension. I asked where that would have come from. "Rage," he said. That stopped me. "I have rage?" "We all have rage," he said. I protested that I didn't feel what I would call rage. He held up a hand. "I've known you a few minutes now. Let me ask you something: You're a good guy, right?" I said I guessed so, tried to be anyway. "No — I mean you need to be a really good guy, right? You want people to see you as a really nice, terrific guy. It's incredibly important to you that you be seen in this world as such a goooood guy. Am I right?" I thought for a second as he held me in a penetrating gaze, and admitted that yes, he might be right there. "Sheeesh," he said. "Lots of rage." With Dr. Sarno's diagnosis relief came quickly, though it would be years before I would more fully comprehend the mind-body connection.

Through this self-examination, I felt pulled to create work that spoke to me. That year, I wrote a novel on the train, with a daily goal of writing one page on the 6:13 am into the city, another on the 6:04 pm home. The resulting "Golden Parachute" is the tale of down-and-out salesman Harry Cathcart, a mid-forties guy who has just figured out the beeline to a loafer's heaven. He'll fake his way into a small company CEO job, and then screw up so badly that his board will be only too happy to send him packing — with a big juicy severance package. Was I projecting? Nonsense!

Transitioning from Life's First Half to the Second

The often uncomfortable — even painful — move from the first half of life into the second is less about the passage of time and more about life as we have lived it and how we reflect on that experience. It is our response to and thinking about what we have done and had done to us that triggers a true transition. Most of us arrive at midlife hauling a mixed bag of triumph and tragedy. Even the most feted or forlorn among us have a nagging sense of things left undone, of life unlived. Most of us choose to ignore this potentially disruptive summons, until ... something happens.

Filmmakers know this intuitively. In most movies, the story really kicks off with an "inciting incident" that shifts or even shatters the seemingly stable world of the hero. Screenwriter Blake Snyder described it this way:

"There is a sense in the set-up that a storm is about to hit, because for things to stay as they are ... is death. Things must change. Telegrams, getting fired, news that you have three days to live, the knock at the door — all can knock down the world as it is. Boom!"

Life-altering events happen to all of us. Serious illness strikes, success at work raises the stakes, a marriage starts to fray, a child leaves home, an unexpected termination stalls a career, or the soul-shattering loss of a loved one is endured. In all of these, the firm ground beneath us quakes and the house around us shivers. Often, what first shows up as suffering brings the most focus. Potentially life-altering questions emerge. For me it was the double-whammy of career interruption with a life-threatening diagnosis.

Suddenly, the future I'd imagined did not seem quite so certain. If it all ended sooner than planned, what would be the verdict on this life — my verdict on my life? If tomorrow evaporates, what was I doing with today? As Hollis asks: "Who am I — aside from the roles that I play and the obligations I fulfill?"

Of course, reactions to events differ. Sincere questioning can be put off, the summons ignored. But the call returns — again and again and again. If we choose to recognize that the call is real, new and pressing questions emerge, all centered around the fundamental question:

"What is the meaning of my life?"

- What has really been happening in my life to this point? Why?

- Whose life have I been leading anyway?

- Why do I seemingly repeat the same patterns over and over?

- What is really true for me, deep down inside — and how can I now bring that out?

In my own life, I learned that it is never too late to heed a summons from the soul. Remember my late teen attraction to television and radio? At 50, and still drawn to write my own stories after having been given a second chance at life, I left corporate environs behind and plunged into a world very different than the one I had called home for three decades.

In what some might see as a clichéd midlife turn, I sought to learn how to write — and specifically for the screen. After reading every how-to book available, a natural next step was to immerse myself in a community of striving creatives that saw this as more than a frivolous distraction.

In my 50s, I enrolled in Columbia University's MFA program for film. Jumping into the most collaborative experience of my life, I was able to partake in experiences my previous careerist self could not have imagined — writing, directing and producing six short films, and writing three feature-length screenplays. While at Columbia I also had the unexpected fun of being cast in 26 short films (mostly due to physical attributes that my twenty-something classmates had not yet developed — my silvery mane chief among them). I thought those windows had closed for me long ago, that those dreams would have to wait for another life, maybe in another dimension. I was wrong, and happily so.

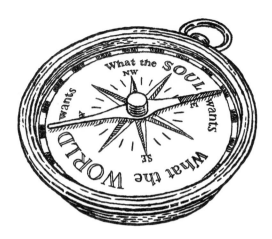

New Life in the Second Half: Unexpected Blossoms

We began by citing the core concern of the first half of life — discovering and then striving to live up to what we think the world expects of us. Our turn into the second half — be it traumatic or relatively tranquil — opens the possibility for living beyond the expectations of others. According to Hollis, the core question here can shift to "What does the soul want of me?" Age has brought us a gift with this chance to rethink and reset. What am I here for anyway? What and who do I really love? What is the unique contribution that I can make in the days and years remaining to me? What is it that wants to be brought into the world through me?

Struggle, scars or emergent wisdom have helped us see the drivers of the first half more clearly for what they were — necessary perhaps, but not sufficient for the rest of the journey. Those things we once wanted so badly — the top job, the BMW, the kitchen worthy of a magazine — are found perhaps to be nice (don't get me wrong), but have fallen short in providing enduring contentment and happiness.

Midlife can be a time of struggle and crisis — but can lead to unforeseen growth and joy. The potential exists for the character and course of the days to be deeper and richer than what was experienced before. New beginnings in the second half often start as faint signals, an intimation of something different just over the horizon. They can manifest as an idea, an impression, or even an image. True change usually requires more than a new address or some other outer change. Genuine beginnings depend on internal alignment rather than external shifts.

Here are a few ways that the second half of life can differ from the first:

THE FIRST HALF OF LIFE	THE SECOND HALF OF LIFE
Formation of a Strong Ego	Development of Conscience
Acquiring/Status/Success	Contributing/Significance
Knowledge	Wisdom
What the world expects of me	What the soul wants of me
Religion/Dogma	Personal Spirituality
Considerate of Outside Authority	Recovery of Personal Authority
Ambition/Performance	Inspiration/Meaning
Happiness is out there	Happiness is inside me
Competition/Scarcity	Cooperation/Abundance
Control	Acceptance/Forgiveness
Fear/Driven	Love/Inspired

Working through the many transitions — large and small — that collectively usher us from the first half to the potentialities of the second half is itself a process. Understanding the nature of transition and embracing the skills of flourishing can support our intention of living fully in the second half of life. We can:

- Forge a more meaningful path centered on purpose and relationship, while consigning our first half-focus on security and acceptance to the rearview mirror.

- Stop craving success as defined by others, opting instead for significance in contribution to others.

- See more clearly the patterns and voices that moved our first half, and release them, choosing conscious priorities and behaviors for our second half.

- Cease our deferral to those who "know what we should be/do," and recover personal authority — to find what is true for ourselves and live it in the world (Hollis).

- Reach back and forward to rediscover aspects of ourselves left behind or hidden away in our first-half agenda — and grasp the part of our lives yet to be lived.

- Look less "out there" for something or someone who will fix our lives, and grasp fully that our solutions lie within.

- Focus less on intense competition in a world defined by scarcity, and embrace cooperation to create abundance for ourselves and others.

- Move from being driven by ambition and fear to becoming inspired by meaning and love.

Ideas to Consider — Transitioning to the Second Half of Life

- Resist the siren call to stay where you are in some seemingly comfortable spot. Embark on a journey of growth and adventure. Relegate security to the rearview mirror, seeking an even more meaningful life, contributing perhaps to an even larger community.

- Be alert for the "Call to Adventure" — the inciting incident that signals the possibility for meaningful change and growth — even when brought on by suffering.

- Be aware of these ways of ignoring the summons to change:

   Doubling down on what worked before.

   Chasing after that certain something new that will solve everything — a new partner, new house, new car, new job, new body.

   Looking for solace in a variety of addictions — to work, alcohol, drugs, shopping, television, even exercise.*

- Strive to become more conscious about what has driven past choices and patterns, and what forces are acting on today's choices.

- Practice the 13 skills of happiness you are about to read about. Each of the skills leads to greater resilience in the face of setbacks and to a deeper, more meaningful, rewarding and joyful second half of life.

*Source: "Finding Meaning in the Second Half of Life," James Hollis

Quotes About the Second Half of Life

1. "In the middle of the journey of our life, I found myself within a dark wood where the straight way was lost."

—DANTE ALIGHIERI

2. "To be yourself in a world that is constantly trying to make you something else is the greatest accomplishment."

—RALPH WALDO EMERSON

3. "We cannot live the afternoon of life according to the program of life's morning — for what was great in the morning will be little at evening, and what in the morning was true will at evening become a lie."

—CARL JUNG

4. "Too long in exile. Too long not singing my song."

—VAN MORRISON

5. "Rock bottom became the solid foundation on which I rebuilt my life."

—J.K. ROWLING

6. *"If you can see your path laid out in front of you step by step, you know it's not your path. Your own path you make with every step you take. That's why it's your path."*

—JOSEPH CAMPBELL

7. *"People spend years commuting long distances to work long hours at jobs they hate, just to buy stuff they don't need to impress people they don't like."*

—NIGEL MARSH

8. *"Telegrams, getting fired, news you have three days to live, a knock at the door — all knock down the world as it is. Boom! It's the opposite of good news, and yet, by the time the adventure is over, it's what leads the hero to happiness."*

—BLAKE SNYDER

9. *"Defeat strips away false values and makes you realize what you really want. It stops you from chasing butterflies and puts you to work digging for gold."*

—WILLIAM MOULTON MARSTON

10. *"The task of the first half is to build the container. The task of the second is to find the actual contents the container was meant to hold."*

—RICHARD ROHR

11. "The greatest burden a child can carry is the unlived life of the parent."

—CARL JUNG

12. "In the second half, we move from being driven to being drawn. We were meant to thrive, not just survive."

—RICHARD ROHR

13. "I didn't see it then, but getting fired was the best thing that could have happened to me. The heaviness of being successful was replaced by the lightness of being a beginner again. It freed me to enter one of the most creative periods of my life."

—STEVE JOBS

14. "Sometimes the best light comes from a burning bridge."

—DON HENLEY

15. "Unlike a good soldier, you're going to choose your battles. You can't be tricked into superhuman heroics for someone else's dream anymore."

—BARBARA SHER

16. "Remember you have two lives. You get your second life when you realize you have only one."

—FRANK LIDDY

17. "We don't pay attention to that inner task until we have had some kind of fall or failure in our outer tasks."
—RICHARD ROHR

*18. "Sometimes with
the bones of the black
sticks left when the fire
has gone out*

*someone has written
something new
in the ashes of your life.*

*You are not leaving.
Even as the light fades quickly now,
you are arriving."*
—DAVID WHYTE

19. "If you bring forth what is within you, what you bring forth will save you. If you do not bring forth what is within you, what you do not bring forth will destroy you."
—GOSPEL OF THOMAS

FINDING PEACE
WITH THE PAST

Chapter 3

FORGIVENESS

The weak can never forgive. Forgiveness is the attribute of the strong.

—MAHATMA GANDHI

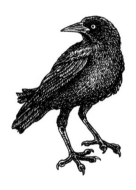

The Skills of Forgiveness

Most of us drift into the second half of life with the blackbird of guilt or anger sitting on our shoulder. We feel remorse over things we did or didn't do, or anger that someone hurt us or prevented us from achieving desired dreams. The accumulation of such feelings binds us to the past, limits our future and prevents us from living in the present. For people who can't forgive or let go of anger or remorse, time does not move forward but repeatedly cycles back to the event that generated these negative feelings.

Forgiveness thus takes on even greater importance in the second half of life, as it liberates us from these feelings of remorse and anger.

The past doesn't really exist. Our only access to it is through our memories. What we carry in our memories, how we choose to remember our past, has a profound effect on our joy in the present. And what we choose to remember we have control over.

Two skills lead to peace with the past: forgiveness and gratitude.

The first, forgiveness, enables us to let go of or diminish hurts of the past. The second, gratitude, enables us to amplify or bring to the forefront good events of the past. The fact that these two skills bring happiness is simple arithmetic. Forgiveness may be the most difficult of the skills, while gratitude is one of the easiest. Let's dig deeper into the skill of forgiveness and why it has such power to change our lives. We'll also explore why it is so difficult to forgive and learn certain tools that facilitate the practice of this powerful skill. We'll deal with gratitude in the next chapter.

I think Gandhi had it right when he wrote: "The weak can never forgive. Forgiveness is the attribute of the strong." Think of the powerful people of the past who were well known for their ability to forgive despite the wrongs perpetrated against them: Gandhi, Abraham Lincoln, Nelson Mandela, Martin Luther King Jr. These people could never have accomplished what they did without their incredible ability to forgive. Without forgiveness, we are forever bound to our past hurts. We relive them over and over in our minds. William Faulkner captured it well when he wrote, "The past is never dead. It's not even past."

Forgiveness, both giving and receiving, is a powerful human experience that can have a profound effect on our ability to flourish.

Let's first recognize that forgiveness is a skill. In fact, it is two very different skills.

The first forgiveness skill is the ability to forgive others. This skill consists of letting go of the desire for vengeance. When someone has hurt us, or we imagine they have hurt us, there is a natural tendency to want to strike back, to hurt them in some way. Forgiveness is the releasing of that feeling, such that we no longer seek revenge. It is not just saying we forgive them, it is actually releasing the desire to act in a spiteful way.

Most of us are probably pretty good at "transactional forgiveness," where we confront the person who has harmed us, they confess and apologize, and we more or less emerge triumphant and unburdened of anger. What is a lot more difficult, but essential to flourishing, is "unconditional forgiveness" — forgiving those who do not show contrition or remorse. Unconditional forgiveness is what makes forgiveness such a difficult skill. Most of us wait for the other person to deserve our forgiveness. This is a mistake. We should practice unconditional forgiveness not because others deserve it, but because we deserve it. We are the beneficiary.

Anger can serve an important purpose: to ensure others respect our needs and desires. But carrying anger, once it has served its purpose, is destructive. Anger is one of the most prevalent emotions Americans experience. It's estimated that over 40% of us are perpetually angry, even though anger is extremely toxic to our health, raising our risk of heart disease and cancer.

Most of us tend to hold on to and keep close all our little grudges like cherished pets, even though they do not serve us well. One reason we hold on to anger is because it is a complex emotion that elicits both pleasure and pain. The pain is associated with the event that hurt us. The pleasure is derived from a feeling of self-righteousness and the contemplation of payback.

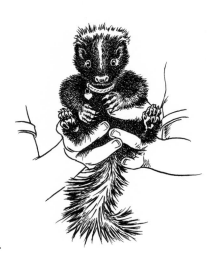

Choosing to forgive someone is choosing to focus on their goodness rather than their faults. It's a liberating skill in that it releases us from anger, resentment and hate.

The second forgiveness skill is the forgiveness of self. This is a skill of self-esteem. Forgiving of self requires that we learn from the mistakes we have made, seek atonement, change our behavior and then release the feelings of remorse and guilt. It is believing that we are worthy of forgiveness and worthy of happiness. Like all negative emotions, remorse and guilt have a very real purpose. They help us change our harmful behavior. But once they have fulfilled that purpose, continuing to feel guilt can be harmful and detrimental to our happiness.

You can be good at one of these skills and lousy at the other, good at both or lousy at both. I am not sure there is a lot of correlation between the two skills. In general, I find women have difficulty forgiving themselves, but are better at forgiving others. This is borne out in research suggesting women are somewhat less self-compassionate than men. It seems men are great at forgiving themselves but lousy at forgiving others.

There are only four things you can do with hurts from the past:

1. **You can forget them.** It's great if that happens, but many of the hurts we experience or cause are hard to forget.

2. **We can repress them,** or tell ourselves to forget them, but they always seem to come back in insidious ways.

3. **We can hold on to them.** This is the choice we often make, a choice that makes achieving happiness difficult.

4. **We can forgive ourselves and others.** This is the only voluntary choice we have that leads to happiness.

People often think that by forgiving someone we are being soft, or that we are inviting that person back into our lives. Not so. If you are in an abusive relationship, get out of the relationship, set boundaries and then forgive. There is nothing passive about forgiveness. Forgiveness is an act of courage, not cowardice.

I used to suggest that forgiveness was like Tide detergent: "It gets the dirt out." I have come to think that this is too simplistic. The truth is that it doesn't get the dirt out. Forgiveness enables us to integrate the hurts — either hurts we have caused or experienced — into our lives so that we grow and learn from the experiences, accepting them as part of who we are and allowing us to move on. The hurts we have inflicted or endured become part of the myriad experiences that make up who we are, and through the acceptance of these hurts, we become deeper and more resilient.

You, me ... we are all a combination of highs and lows, good and bad, sinner and saint. It is through forgiving ourselves that we come to accept our darkness while moving toward our light. And in forgiving others, we accept their darkness and focus on their light.

How to Practice Forgiveness

In practicing forgiveness of others, it is probably most helpful to realize that the key beneficiary of forgiveness is the person forgiving, not the person forgiven. The anger we carry around toward someone who has harmed us hurts us far more than the person toward whom we direct that anger. Forgiveness is a gift we give ourselves.

Here are several tools for better practicing forgiveness of self and others:

1. REACH Process: Everett L. Worthington, author of several books on forgiveness, has a process he calls the REACH process of forgiveness. Here's how it works:

- **Recall:** Recall the event.

- **Empathize:** Empathize with the person who has transgressed (either someone else or yourself). Try to put yourself in their shoes or your shoes at that particular point in time … there may have been extenuating circumstances. Try to understand why they/you might have caused this hurt.

- **Altruism:** Give the altruistic gift of forgiveness.

- **Commit:** Commit some act to confirm the forgiveness (write a letter, make a phone call, etc.)

- **Hold On:** Hold on to the act of forgiveness such that when you start to feel anger or remorse, remind yourself that you have forgiven.*

*Source: "Forgiving and Reconciling: Bridges to Wholeness & Hope," Everett L. Worthington

2. Stop looking for things to be offended by. In fact, see if you can become the person who is almost never offended. You can stick up for yourself, without being offended, and doing so is beneficial to your relationships and your health. Have the attitude, "I have control over how I choose to feel and I choose to feel peaceful regardless of how someone else treats me."

3. The three R's (Recognize, Recompense, Release): To admit we have erred and be responsible for the consequences is the first step toward wisdom and the only path to release. Guilt binds us to the past, destroying our ability to move forward and limiting our joy in the present. These three R's are the basis of the process of confession.

4. Consider how others have forgiven: When Nelson Mandela left Robben Island after being imprisoned for 27 years, he said if he continued to hate those who had held him captive, he would still be in prison. His forgiveness enabled South Africa to move on. Conversely, Zimbabwe, just to the north of South Africa, was founded more on revenge or retribution than forgiveness. It has struggled mightily as a result. If Nelson Mandela can forgive having been wrongly imprisoned for 27 years, surely, we can find a way to forgive what has happened to us.

5. Grace: If you have trouble forgiving yourself for a past behavior that you have long since changed, consider Paul Tillich's definition of grace: "Accept the fact that you are accepted, despite the fact that you are unacceptable." If the remorse you feel no longer serves a useful purpose, see if you can release it and move on.

Reflections for the Second Half

- Are you better at forgiving yourself or forgiving others?

- Identify one or two things you carry concerning remorse or anger. How long and how often have you experienced these feelings? How do these feelings affect you and those around you?

- Are there things you've done or thought that you believe won't be forgiven?

- What steps might you take to move beyond these negative emotions?

Quotes About Forgiveness

1. *"You only have to forgive once. To resent, you have to do it all day, every day. You have to keep remembering all the bad things. It's too much work."*
—M.L. STEDMAN, "THE LIGHT BETWEEN OCEANS"

2. *"The past is never dead. It's not even past."*
—WILLIAM FAULKNER

3. *"Conscience is a mother-in-law whose visit never ends."*
—H. L. MENCKEN

4. *"Accept the fact that you are accepted, despite the fact that you are unacceptable."*
—PAUL TILLICH'S DEFINITION OF "GRACE"

5. *"I am resolved never again to hold rancor, however justified, towards a group of people, whatever their race, religion, convictions, prejudices or error."*
—IRÈNE NÉMIROVSKY, RUSSIAN NOVELIST LIVING IN FRANCE, BEFORE HER DEATH IN AUSCHWITZ IN 1942

6. *"As I walked out the door toward the gate that would lead to my freedom, I knew if I didn't leave my bitterness and hatred behind, I'd still be in prison."*

—NELSON MANDELA

7. *"We remember so we can have roses in winter. Unfortunately, we also remember so we can be up agitated at 2:00 a.m. and angry about something that happened half a lifetime ago."*
—DOUGLAS A. SMITH

8. *"The paradox of vengefulness is that it makes men dependent upon those who have harmed them, believing that their release from pain will come only when their tormentors suffer."*
—LAURA HILLENBRAND, "UNBROKEN"

9. *"When you hold resentment toward another, you are bound to that person or condition by an emotional link that is stronger than steel. Forgiveness is the only way to dissolve that link and get free."*
—CATHERINE PONDER

10. *"Resentment is like taking poison and waiting for the other person to die."*
—UNKNOWN

11. *"Hakuna Matata" (Put your past behind you)*
— FROM "THE LION KING"

Chapter 4

GRATITUDE

Gratitude is not only the greatest of virtues but the parent of all others.

—MARCUS TULLIUS CICERO

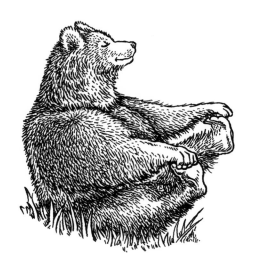

The Skill of Gratitude

Aging makes many of us increasingly aware of how blessed we are. Even so, we still often focus on what we don't have, what we've been denied. Our second half of life can be greatly enhanced when we stop thinking about what we don't have, focus on what we do have and choose to live with a sense of gratitude.

Gratitude is probably the easiest of the 13 skills that lead to flourishing to practice. It is also foundational to all the other skills we will discuss. Those who live with gratitude almost by definition are happy and those who live without gratitude most likely find it very hard to be happy. Each day we can choose to live with gratitude, or we can choose to live with a sense of entitlement or anger. One choice leads to happiness, the other does not. Importantly, the choice is ours.

Gratitude is big-picture thinking. Entitlement is small-picture thinking. Let me explain. I like to play golf. I am not very good, but most days I enjoy it. Someone once joked, "In golf, bad shots come in series of threes, so a fourth bad shot is the beginning of a new series." Well, by the time I am into my second series, I sometimes become more than a little angry. But if I take a moment and reflect on the bigger picture, I can often get myself in a better place.

The big picture is that I am physically able to walk and play golf. I am outside on a nice day. I am with friends. I can afford to play golf ... there are so many things to be thankful for while playing golf. And if I step even further back, I realize I have a wonderful wife, two great sons, a wonderful daughter-in-law and a cute, spunky little granddaughter. And big, big picture, I have been given the gift of life. Gratitude is big-picture thinking.

We often take our gifts for granted, as if we are simply entitled to all these things. By taking them for granted, we miss the opportunity to practice the easiest and most foundational skill, the skill of gratitude.

When I get aggravated about something around the house that needs fixing — a leaky faucet, a running toilet, faulty WiFi — my wife reminds me, "You have rich boy problems." She is right (as usual). As Jane Parker of VivaLaMe points out, there are real problems that others are confronting every day: 22,000 children die each day because of poverty, 1 billion children worldwide live in poverty, 750 million people do not have access to clean drinking water, 1.6 billion people live without electricity and nearly 1 billion people do not have enough food to eat.

Again big-picture thinking brings me back to feeling grateful for what I have and who I am. Feeling entitled is debilitating. We think we are entitled to good health, a good job, a good life. In truth, we are entitled to nothing. When we think we are entitled and we face adversity or a setback, we easily default to passivity, whining and anger. We fail to pursue the work and struggle to realize our hopes and dreams. Gratitude brings happiness for a very simple reason: It brings the good things in our lives to the forefront of our minds. It magnifies the good. Just like forgiveness minimizes negatives, gratitude adds positives to our lives.

Positive psychologists have conducted experiments to measure the impact gratitude has on happiness. They split volunteers into two groups. Participants in the first group were asked to write whatever they chose at the end of each day. Participants in the second group were asked to record three things for which they were grateful at the end of each day, and, if they had time, why they were grateful for these things. At the end of 30 days, the positive psychologists measured the happiness of the two groups. The group that wrote about what they were grateful for were measurably happier than the other group. Given even more time to keep their journals, the happiness levels between the two groups widened.

We miss a hundred — no, probably a thousand — opportunities a day to express our gratitude. That this world exists and that we exist within it are incredible miracles beyond even our comprehension. The problem is we take it all for granted. We are spoiled. All these beautiful gifts no longer move us, no longer bring us happiness. We don't even notice. Just another sunrise, another wind gust rustling the leaves, another full moon, another child's smile ... so what? No big deal. Miracles are happening around us every second and we don't even notice. Rather, what we notice is the spilled cup of coffee, the driver who cuts us off, the WiFi that is a little slower than we would like.

When we move positive experiences and thoughts to the front of our awareness it raises our sense of gratitude. Journaling is a great way to do this. Here is an entry in my journal after I climbed the mountain behind our home in the Adirondack Region of upstate New York several years ago. Each time I read this, it brings back to me the sense of joy and peace I felt on that day.

It is late October 2008. Last night it snowed at the higher elevations, leaving the mountain tops around the lake white and the shoulders of the mountains still alive with fall colors of orange, red and yellow. I was supposed to leave early this morning, but when I awoke, with the sun rising over the mountains on the eastern shore, I felt drawn to hike to the top of White Pine Mountain and look down at the grandeur of it all.

As I walked up the mining road, abandoned now for almost 100 years, an errant cloud dropped snow on me and the trail before me, even as the sun shone brightly in the east. The snow made not a sound, but somehow it seemed to fill all my senses. When I reached the top and looked down at Black Mountain, 20 miles to the south, I felt an incredible level of peace. I wanted to change nothing, even myself. I felt I belonged here at this moment as much as the mountains, trees, lake and sky that surrounded me.

I reach down and gather several leaves, I suppose to remind me of this moment. I run my hands over the lichen and the moss that cover the rock upon which I am sitting. I bend further down and smell the mustiness of the rock and lichen. I wonder how long this rock and lichen have stood here and kept watch over it all. I just wonder.

Shortly, I must leave. I look back one more time and ponder when I will next return. I want to hold on to this moment, for time to stop for just a little while, but alas it is not to be. I turn and begin the walk back down the mountain, holding on to the fading sense of peace and wonder. I know I will return. —DAS, October 30, 2008

People often think circumstances dictate our gratitude. Not so. The same circumstances that lead to gratitude from one person can elicit anger from another. It is less about the circumstances than the perspective. It is difficult to be happy without being grateful. Without gratitude, we focus on the negative. We see ourselves as victims and limit our effectiveness and attractiveness to those around us. Misery may like company, but guess what ... company does not like misery. Victims don't make great friends.

Gratitude leads to more satisfaction with life. It enables us to be more resilient, more social and outward-focused, more optimistic. The Internet has made us experts at comparing ourselves to others and counting their blessings. We need to return to counting our own blessings.

How to Practice Gratitude

1. Choose your channel: Every morning you have the choice to turn to the gratitude channel or the entitlement channel. Taking a few moments before you get up to express the things you are grateful for is a wonderful way to start the day "on the right side of the bed." I have a simple little tool I use each morning to turn myself to the gratitude channel. When I wake up I stick my left foot out from under the covers, and if I don't see a toe tag, I rejoice and know it is going to be a great day!

2. Tell others you are grateful: Write three emails each morning to people at work or in your personal life who you want to thank for helping you.

3. Keep a gratitude journal: At the end of each day,

write down three things you are grateful for. Your journal will be even more impactful if you take the time to write why you are grateful. For instance, if you are grateful for your wife or son, explain why you are grateful. If you keep this up for at least four weeks, I guarantee you will be meaningfully happier.

4. Create a gratitude gallery: Take a picture of something you are grateful for each week and keep the photos on your phone in a "gratitude gallery." When you feel a little blue, pull out the gallery and look through the photos.

5. Go for a gratitude walk. If you like to walk for exercise, as you walk just start listing things you are grateful for … "I am grateful for the sky, the trees, the clouds, that I can walk, I can see, hear, speak, for my family, my home, my friends …" You could probably walk several miles and not run out of things to be grateful for.

6. Capture your memories: When an experience brings you great joy — a wonderful hike, a great family vacation, a time alone that brought you remarkable peace — find a way to capture it. Write about it, take photos, bring back something that reminds you of the time and keeps the memory fresh.

7. Set a daily objective: This is a wonderful Buddhist concept known as "One at the beginning and one at the end." Basically, it's starting the morning with a statement of how we want the day to unfold, such as, "May I not speak or act out of anger today," or "May I act with kindness when challenged today." At the end of the day, review how the day went and how you did, including where you have succeeded and where you have come up short. Do this without judgment or being hard on yourself, while recognizing what a gift it is to be able to acknowledge what has happened without denial.

Reflections for the Second Half

- How often do you experience gratitude?

- What actions might you take to increase these feelings of gratitude?

- How might you start and end your day to experience more gratitude?

- What things prevent you from feeling gratitude and what might you do about those things so you feel more gratitude?

Quotes About Gratitude

1. *"Joy is the simplest form of gratitude."*
—KARL BARTH

2. *"So much has been given to me I have not time to ponder over that which has been denied."*
—HELEN KELLER

3. *"There are only two ways to live your life. One is as though nothing is a miracle. The other is as though everything is a miracle."*
—ALBERT EINSTEIN

4. *"To see a World in a Grain of Sand
And a Heaven in a Wild Flower
Hold Infinity in the palm of your hand
And Eternity in an hour."*
—WILLIAM BLAKE, "AUGURIES OF INNOCENCE"

5. *"Gratitude is not only the greatest of virtues, but the parent of all the others."*
—MARCUS TULLIUS CICERO

6. *"Beauty seen makes the one who sees it more beautiful."*
—DAVID STEINDL-RAST, "A LISTENING HEART"

7. *"Our planet is a prodigious miracle, a unique happening in billions of years of evolution, in eons of light years of space. We will never cherish it enough. We will never be grateful enough. This miracle should be the object of constant joy, love and admiration."*

—ROBERT MULLER

8. *"I can't tell you anything that, in a few minutes, will tell you how to be rich. But I can tell you how to feel rich, which is far better, let me tell you first-hand, than being rich. Be grateful ... it is the only totally reliable get-rich-quick scheme."*

—BEN STEIN

9. *"We would give almost anything for what we already have."*

—TONY HOAGLAND

10. *"Quod cupio mecum est." (What I want, I already have.)*

—OVID'S "METAMORPHOSES" AND STENCILED ON A FRIEND'S KITCHEN WALL IN VERMONT

HAVING CONFIDENCE IN THE FUTURE

Chapter 5

FOFO — FAITH, OPTIMISM, FLEXIBILITY AND OPENNESS

When one door of happiness closes, another opens;
but often we look so long at the closed door that we
do not see the one which has been opened for us.
—HELEN KELLER

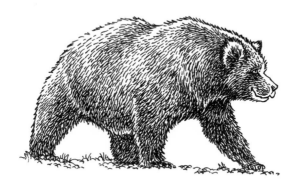

The challenges we face in the second half of life are often more significant than the ones we faced earlier. Bigger challenges require better skills for handling them effectively. This chapter on having confidence in the future, and the next on resilience, will better enable you to flourish, even in the face of difficult, unexpected and undesired challenges.

Here is the premise that underlies this chapter: Much of our unhappiness in life is due to our rigid and fixed concept about how the future should evolve and our resulting inability to adjust to the inevitable diversions the universe takes as the future unfolds.

How we perceive the future can have a profound impact on our ability to flourish. People who live with joy recognize they play a significant role in shaping the future, even if they don't control it. They believe that if they do their part, the universe will do its part by bringing them what they need, if not necessarily what they want. They focus on what they can do to prepare and then they accept and adjust to whatever diversions the future brings. They live with faith, optimism, flexibility and openness — something I call FOFO.

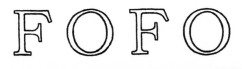

Faith. Optimism. Flexibility. Openness.

My oldest son Gordon helped me understand and better practice FOFO. Gordon is mentally challenged because of oxygen deficiency at birth. For years, I agonized about Gordon's future. I worried he would never be able to walk, until he walked. I worried he would never be able to speak, until he spoke. I worried he would never go to school, until he did. I agonized about every aspect of his future. With time, I've come to realize that what I really agonized about was MY future, how it would affect me.

Sometime around his middle teenage years, I started to think about Gordon differently. I began to realize that Gordon was a great son just the way he was. What he lacked in IQ, he more than made up for in EQ, or emotional intelligence. I started to focus on what he could do as opposed to what he couldn't do. I came to realize that I couldn't have a more wonderful oldest son. He is an incredible blessing to me; my dear wife Phyllis; and our other son Greg, who is on the other end of the intellectual spectrum and an equal blessing in our lives. If I had embraced FOFO earlier, I would have spared myself years of agonizing. Now don't get me wrong — adjusting to the realization that one's son or daughter is mentally handicapped is something that takes significant time, but doing so should not have taken me 10 to 15 years!

Faith

The first thing I needed to be at peace with Gordon's future, and my own, was faith. The word "faith" corresponds to the Greek noun "pistis" meaning to trust, to have confidence, to be reliable. Without faith, when we experience difficulty, our minds conjure up all kinds of negative scenarios about the future. As I've found, imagination without faith is a cruel master.

Faith is a belief about the future that stands without evidence, making faith a very personal individual matter. In childhood and early adulthood, most of us have lots of people (usually parents) and institutions (particularly religious institutions) that influence what we believe, that shape our faith. As the second half of life unfolds, our faith often takes on a more personal perspective as we put less stock in outer authority and begin to gradually develop our own internal authority.

My own faith is reflective of this. I was raised a Christian and, while I consider myself a Christian today, I would venture that many of my beliefs are not fully consistent with what I was taught in Sunday school or what gets preached on Sunday mornings. One of my beliefs that is consistent with Christianity is love. At the foundation of my faith, of everything I believe, is "love." In fact, I believe love is the foundation of all valid religions and of successful living. If I could consistently act with love — care for self, care for others and care for place, for the world we all inhabit — my actions would benefit me and everyone with whom I interact. All of the skills covered in this book — forgiveness, kindness, gratitude, optimism, relationships, abundance, etc. — are founded on love.

So if faith is essential to confidence in the future, how do we develop it? I think we do this through reflection, through silence, through study, through contemplation, through trial and error. We develop faith by opening our minds and hearts to new perspectives on things that cannot be proven and can only be understood at a deeper level. I also believe faith is more about connection than it is about dogma or doctrine. Having faith connects us to something larger than we are, it enables us to see ourselves as part of a larger whole, to see beyond the immediate difficulties that may surround us — difficulties that would overwhelm us without faith.

Research indicates that many kinds of faith and secular life philosophies can lead to a happiness advantage.

What I think is key is that as we develop faith we begin to find our own answers to difficult, but important questions: Why am I here? What do I value? What do I believe? How do I deal with the setbacks in my life? What is God's role, if any, in my life? When we have faith we come to believe that no matter what happens, perhaps with God's help, we will be able to deal with it.

As with most skills that lead to flourishing, faith is something we find within ourselves. It's an inner source of courage and a sense of hope that can sustain us in times of turmoil. Discovering and developing our own unique faith is a key task in the second half of life, since what makes a profound difference in our lives is less what happens to us than how we respond to what happens. If our inner lives, our beliefs and our deepest values remain uncharted territory, we will never develop the courage and tenacity needed to face the tragedies we all invariably face. In turmoil and adversity we learn, as the Buddhists say, "to coax the lotus from the mud." Faith makes us far more resilient and it is therefore the first skill that enables us to face the future with confidence.

Optimism

The second thing I needed as Gordon was growing up was "optimism." Optimism is the degree to which we expect favorable outcomes to occur. Optimism and happiness correlate almost one to one. Optimism is the mirror image of gratitude. Grateful people see good things in their past and optimists see good things in their future. Optimism fuels our movement toward living with joy.

Looking at the bright side of things is not naive, unless

we use it as an excuse for not preparing for the future. Often people think that pessimism prepares us better for the future, that we are more prepared to deal with setbacks. Research shows just the opposite. People who are more optimistic do better with setbacks. Here's why: When we encounter a setback in life and we are thinking optimistically, we make the setback temporary, specific to the event and controllable. If a student fails a test and is thinking optimistically, he might say to himself, "I shouldn't have gone to the party the night before the exam; I should have studied harder. I have a history test next week. If I study for it, I will do just fine." When we are thinking pessimistically, we tend to make setbacks permanent, pervasive and uncontrollable. If a student fails a test and is thinking pessimistically, he might think, "I am so stupid!"

Thinking optimistically broadens our thinking and opens us to new solutions to the challenges we face. Yes, you can be too optimistic and misuse this skill, but in general, being optimistic leads to happiness.

There is a clear connection between what you expect and how your life unfolds. Psychologists call this phenomenon "confirmation bias." When we think pessimistically, we look for things in our environment that "confirm" that negative bias. Conversely, when we think optimistically, we look for things that "confirm" our positive bias. In other words, our perception shapes our world. As Anaïs Nin said, "We don't see things as they are, we see things as we are."

Martin Seligman began his career with the study of what he called "learned helplessness." Through his research, he found that when people experience uncontrollable negative events many become passive and give up trying to do anything to overcome their predicament. They learn to be helpless. But not everyone becomes helpless. From Seligman's perspective, about 10% of the people he studied became helpless "at the drop of a hat," yet about one-third of the people who came to his laboratory never became helpless. They kept trying to find solutions to the challenges he gave them. What was the distinguishing characteristic? It was optimism. Seligman found those who refused to be helpless had a habit of saying, "It's temporary; it's just one situation and there is something I can do about it."*

How we look to the future affects the quality of our lives. Here is how psychologists Christopher Peterson and Edward Chang put it: "Optimism, however measured, is linked to desirable characteristics — happiness, perseverance, achievement and health — while pessimism is associated with undesirable characteristics such as helplessness, unhappiness, poor health and not trying to cope with difficulties."**

There is a role for pessimism in our lives. When you are driving on a cold winter day after a snowstorm, you want to envision what might happen if you encounter a patch of ice and so you drive accordingly. Most of the time, however, we do better when our predominant perspective is positive and optimistic.

Optimism is a skill that can be learned. If you struggle with being optimistic, Martin Seligman has written a helpful book called "Learned Optimism: How to Change Your Mind and Your Life."

*Source: "Flourish: Positive Psychology and Positive Interventions" by Martin Seligman, delivered at The University of Michigan, October 7, 2010

**Source: The Resiliency Advantage: Master Change, Thrive Under Pressure, and Bounce Back from Setbacks, by Al Seibert.

Flexibility & Openness

The next two skills I needed were "flexibility" and "openness." First, let's consider flexibility.

When we face the future, most of us look ahead and think about where we want to go and how to get there. We construct an imaginary pathway forward that will take us to that desired future. This is healthy, it gets us to move in the direction of our desired future. The issue is that we tend to see only one pathway forward. We lock onto this pathway. The future will almost always be different than we anticipate. Without the skill of flexibility, as soon as the future begins to unfold in a different way than we planned, we tend to get angry or upset.

What we need is the flexibility to realize there are numerous pathways to take us where we want to go. Rather than get upset, we need to have the flexibility to find new pathways forward that will get us to where we initially wished to be. We need to be able to continually course correct.

The Eagle landed on the moon only a few feet from where it was intended, but it was off course well over 90% of the flight. It was through constant course correction that it landed successfully. So it is with us. Our plans, all plans, are a fixed picture of the future. Nature, by definition, is anything but fixed. Nature is unpredictable, haphazard, varied, diverse ... mysterious. As my college art teacher would tell me, "Straight lines don't exist in nature."

Finally, let's discuss openness. Sometimes we will never get to exactly where we wish to go. There are things in life we must learn to accept. Being open to new destinations and situations we cannot change is an important skill in dealing effectively with the future. If I was still hung up on my oldest son Gordon being the son I envisioned before he was born, I would miss so much of the joy he has to offer to so many who know him. Who knew he would be such a blessing in our lives, just as is our second son Greg? When we are forced to deal with situations that are different than we expected, we can either lament that it is not what we originally envisioned or we can come to see the beauty in our new situation.

How to Practice Faith, Optimism, Flexibility and Openness

In the next chapter on resilience, we provide a number of tools for becoming more resilient, but here are two tools for facing the future with confidence.

1. Good news, bad news, who knows? There is an old Sufi tale about a peasant who exchanges all his worldly possessions for a beautiful stallion. All his neighbors come to tell him, "What great news!" To which he responds, "Good news, bad news, who knows?" That night his stallion runs away and all the neighbors come by to say, "What terrible news!" To which he responds, "Good news, bad news, who knows?" A week later the stallion comes back with 12 mares and all the neighbors say, "What great news!" to which he responds, "Good news, bad news, who knows?" His son goes out to break the horses and falls and breaks his leg, to which the neighbors and the father give the same responses. The King calls all the young men up for battle and the son can't go because of his injury; all the other young men are killed. By now you get the idea. The key message of this tale is to stop judging the things that happen as the future unfolds and instead figure out how to best deal with what happens. We don't actually know if many of the things that happen are good news or bad news. Events considered undesirable — a lost job, a broken marriage, a major health challenge — just might lead to all kinds of new opportunities. How we handle them is often what makes them good or bad news.

2. The PAL system: I have a tool that I'm sure I borrowed from someone, I just don't know who. I call it my PAL system. It goes like this: I Plan, I Act according to that plan, I Learn from what happens, and then return to planning. I try to follow this three-step process.

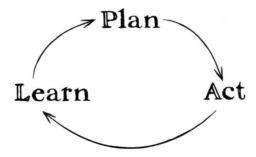

The tough part of staying on the PAL path is this: When we plan and act and things don't turn out as expected, instead of learning and planning again, we get off this path and head over to "Pity City." When my son Gordon was born, I not only went to Pity City, I moved there and became the city's mayor. In moving off the PAL path, we make ourselves a victim. As a friend is fond of telling me, "You can visit Pity City, you just can't move there."

Reflections for the Second Half

- As you look to the future, what are the dominant feelings you have ... excitement, challenge, hope, fear?

- When have you been most confident about the future? When least? Why?

- What changes would you like to make in how you see the future?

Quotes About Having Confidence in the Future

1. *"Whatever is flexible and loving will tend to grow. Whatever is rigid and blocked will wither and die."*
—LAO-TZU

2. *"I never saw a pessimistic general win a battle."*
—GENERAL DWIGHT EISENHOWER

3. *"If you can see your path laid out in front of you step by step, you know it's not your path. Your own path you make with every step you take. That's why it's your path."*
—JOSEPH CAMPBELL

4. *"Pessimism is a shortcut to disappointment."*
—UNKNOWN

5. *"I tend to judge everything and everyone that comes before me. If I would release this judgment and accept others as they are and accept whatever the future presents, I think I would be ever so much happier."*
—DOUGLAS A. SMITH

6. *"Optimism is true moral courage."*
—SIR ERNEST SHACKLETON

7. *"We take any information we receive as confirmation of our mental models. If we have a negative mental model, we look for negative events to confirm that model."*

—DOUGLAS A. SMITH

8. *"No pessimist ever discovered the secret of the stars, or sailed to an uncharted land, or opened a new doorway for the human spirit."*

—HELEN KELLER

9. *"If we could only find the courage to leave our destiny to chance, to accept the fundamental mystery of our lives, then we might be closer to the sort of happiness that comes with innocence."*

—LUIS BUÑUEL

10. *"The future is not someplace we are going, but one we are creating. The paths are not to be found but made. And the activity of making them changes both the maker and the destination."*

—JOHN SCHAAR

11. "The very little engine looked up and saw the tears in the dolls' eyes. And she thought of the good little boys and girls on the other side of the mountain who would not have any toys or good food unless she helped. Then she said, 'I think I can. I think I can.'"

—WATTY PIPER (ARNOLD MUNK),
"THE LITTLE ENGINE THAT COULD"

Chapter 6

RESILIENCE

The things in life that really hurt spare no one.
—DAN BAKER

William H. McRaven, a former Navy SEAL and former commander of all U.S. Special Operations, recalls in his book "Make Your Bed" the important lesson of being "sugar-cookied." Being "sugar-cookied" occurred during SEAL training when the officer in charge decided something was wrong with how a trainee had made his bed or that his uniform wasn't perfect. The officer would tell the trainee to go into the surf in uniform, emerge and roll on the beach until he was covered with sand. The trainee would then have to spend the rest of the day in that uniform. It was not a comfortable experience.

Being "sugar-cookied" was often a random event with no real justification for the punishment. That was the point. The exercise was not so much about punishment, but rather to remind trainees that life isn't always fair and that they needed to accept this unfairness and move on. The trainees that couldn't handle being "sugar-cookied" because it was unfair, were the ones that didn't make it through the training to become SEALs.

Dan Baker's book "What Happy People Know" ends with

the story of a woman who walks into a doctor's office. He is about to tell her she has cancer. He opens the conversation with, "I am about to give you a diagnosis that will color the rest of your life." Before the doctor has the chance to give her the diagnosis, she replies, "Then I will choose what color." In dealing with the indignities we all face in life, we each can choose how they color our lives, and that choice, in many ways, determines whether we flourish or languish.

I guess the message of this chapter is this: In the second half of life get used to being "sugar-cookied" and choose wisely how the setbacks you experience "color" your life.

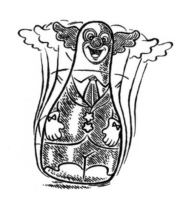

When I was a kid, I had a clown punching bag. I could punch it, and no matter how hard I punched, it always returned to the upright position. I am trying in the second half of my life to be more like that punching bag. No matter what happens to knock me down, I try to bounce back to a sense of well-being. As I write this, I realize I have a lot of work to do in this area. Long term, I think I handle setbacks fairly well, but this isn't until after I have gone through panic, anger, denial, all kinds of destructive phases.

The second half of life brings its own set of challenges. While often painful, these challenges can also be doorways to a richer, more fulfilling life. In this chapter, I want to share ideas on how to become more resilient to successfully meet these challenges. Part of this chapter is devoted to better understanding change and transitions. When major changes occur at any point in our lives, we experience a distinct pattern of stages as we transition. Understanding this pattern and how we feel during each of its stages can help us successfully move through the stages rather than become overwhelmed by them.

Dan Baker has it right, "The things that really hurt in life spare no one." We all experience painful setbacks. No one lives a charmed life — no one. Those of us who seem to be given everything in life make bad decisions that invite pain. Just look at the Hollywood crowd that has fame, fortune and beauty — they often seem to bring pain upon themselves in one form or another.

Because the challenges we face in the second half of life take on greater gravity — such as the loss of parents and other loved ones or our own health-related challenges — knowing how to deal with them effectively, accept them with grace and ultimately rebound is increasingly important.

Often people who experience a major setback in life emerge with what at first glance may seem like a strangely optimistic perspective. Despite their challenge, they may believe that their life is better than it was before the setback. Learning how to adopt that perspective is this chapter's goal.

Our lives begin with loss. We are pushed out of our mother's womb, separated from her heartbeat, and forced into a harsh new world where we begin a lifelong journey of gain and loss, joy and sadness, success and failure. Setbacks are inevitable, so what leads to a flourishing life is not the absence of setbacks, but how we choose to handle the challenges, the hurts, the disappointments, the pain that we all encounter. What sets those who thrive apart from those who don't is resilience. Resilience is defined as "the ability to bend and not break under pressure and then to bounce back." However, in the field of positive psychology, resilience is the ability to not just bounce back, but to experience what is known as "post-traumatic growth."

There are four possible outcomes when we face a crisis. We can become a victim, we can survive, we can recover, or we can thrive and experience post-traumatic growth (PTG).

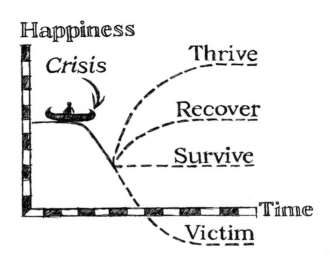

Victims tend to see their fate as determined by forces outside of themselves and to develop what is known as a "vulnerable attributional style." Those who thrive do just the opposite, seeing their fate as something they have power over, developing what is known as a "resilient attributional style." People who thrive also have what psychologist Angela Duckworth calls "grit." She describes grit as "the tendency to pursue long-term goals with passion and persistence." She created a 10-question test called the "Grit Scale" and found West Point cadets who score highest on the scale are more likely to make it through their grueling training. She also tested Chicago public school students, salespeople at a timeshare company and national spelling bee contestants. In each case, the grit scale was better than IQ or talent at predicting success. Hopefully, this chapter enables us to have more grit.

The first step in better dealing with setbacks is changing our perspective on them. Most of us view setbacks as unfavorable. This might seem the right assessment in the short term, but our view might be very different over time. Sometimes, setbacks make our lives better, although this is not immediately evident. Think of the high school sweetheart who dumped you, and when you see them at your 25th high school reunion, you realize they would never have made a good spouse; or the lost job that led to a better career opportunity; or the house you didn't get, only to end up living somewhere else so much better. Setbacks can lead to far better outcomes.

Setbacks serve a very real purpose in our lives. They are not enjoyable, but they are just as important as the good times because they give us perspective and can heighten our appreciation for the good times. We wouldn't know the good times without the bad times, just as we wouldn't know up without down, light without darkness. Good times and bad times are just part of the complex web of life. We can't have the joy of reunion without the pain of farewell, the gift of forgiveness without the pain of remorse or anger. Life is a series of periods of stability followed by periods of instability for everyone and everything. Just as people experience highs and lows, in nature a leaf unfurls and eventually falls, an egg is laid and eventually cracked, a seed blossoms into a flower that eventually fades ... there is no stopping this vacillation.

These periods of instability are full of opportunities to learn and grow. They can draw us closer to God, or if we are not religious, closer to the values and beliefs we hold most dear. While setbacks can be tragic, not capitalizing on the opportunities they present to learn and grow can be equally so. Then the question before us is: How do we move through these periods of instability and turn them into experiences that deepen the meaning in our lives?

Change Versus Transition

I think it is helpful to understand the difference between change and transition. It's often said that people resist change. I think what we resist is not change, so much as the transition that change requires of us.

Change is something that happens. It is an event and it can happen in an instant. Often these changes are beyond our control. We can't resist the change itself any more than we can resist the sun rising tomorrow. What we resist is the transition that is required to successfully deal with the change. Unlike change, transitions take time, often months or years. Let's look more closely at transitions.

I am going to build off the model of transitions by William Bridges from his classic book "Transitions: Making Sense of Life's Changes." Bridges contends that while every transition is unique, every transition is also the same in that it always involves three stages. The first stage is an ending. Something changes. A relationship comes to a close, we are in a job that no longer fills our needs or we lose our job. More tragically, we are diagnosed with a life-threatening illness or lose our spouse to an illness. All these changes require a transition on our part, a letting go.

Endings are almost always difficult. We fear what is unknown, or we deny that we even need to change, or we hang onto something (a relationship, a job) far longer than is appropriate. We hate endings and will often do most anything to avoid them. What we often hate even more is the next phase, the "neutral zone," or what Bridges more accurately calls the "swampland."

The swampland is that time when neither the old nor the new applies. It is a time of discombobulation, disengagement, disorientation ... but it is also a time of discovery. Since we hate the swampland, we often try to jump to the third phase, a beginning, without going through the swampland. We immediately jump to a new job or a new relationship. This is usually a failed strategy, for as Bridges says, "There is no nonstop flight from an ending to a beginning." We simply have to take the time to go through the confusion, the sense of loss that is part of the swampland.

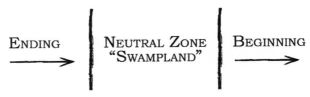

ENDING | NEUTRAL ZONE "SWAMPLAND" | BEGINNING

Source: "Transitions: Making Sense of Life's Changes," William Bridges

Understanding this model is helpful to me, as I hope it is to you. It helps me see that as I face setbacks, the feelings I have of loss, separation, confusion, fear, being adrift are necessary in dealing effectively with the changes and getting to a successful new beginning.

How to Develop Resilience

Here are some ideas to help you successfully move through transitions without becoming a victim:

1. Expect and accept chaos. Chaos is inevitable during change and transition. You simply can't escape the feelings of discombobulation and confusion that come with an ending and crossing the swampland. Rather than agonizing about these feelings, focus on discovering hidden pathways and new perspectives that often emerges from the chaos.

2. Stay in the present. Let go of the "if only" thoughts about the past and the "what if" thoughts about the future. Instead, focus on what you can do now and choose to move forward. Forget about seeking justice, vengeance or blame; it's better to devote energy to moving forward.

3. Act with bravery. I wish there was a substitute for bravery … there isn't. Have the courage to face reality without wallowing in it.

4. Embrace the new you. The loss of a job, a marriage or physical capability can rob us of our identity. Seek a new identity based on the new situation, the new reality.

5. See change and transition not as the ending of what was supposed to be, but perhaps the beginning of what was meant to be. Realize that the life you planned may not be half as beautiful as the new life that lies ahead.

6. Realize you are not the Lone Ranger. Everyone goes through crises. Seek out others who have gone through similar transitions successfully and gain their insights.

7. Dig no holes … at least no deep holes. If you are smoking a pack of cigarettes a day, stop. If you are breaking major commitments to others, stop. Be sure your actions aren't making your situation worse.

8. Continue to care for yourself. Often when challenged, we stop doing the very things that have kept us centered. If you have been exercising regularly, eating well, getting enough sleep, meditating, be sure to keep these routines intact as you head through a transition.

9. Practice telling "redemptive stories." Those who thrive tell stories about how the challenges they faced helped them grow. Such stories are empowering. Victims do just the opposite. They tell "contaminant stories," that suggest their life has been permanently damaged and there is nothing they can do about it. These stories are incredibly self-defeating. Here is a redemptive story: "The jerk fired me, but you know, it opened me up to a whole new exciting career." Here is a contaminant story: "The jerk fired me and my career has been ruined."

10. Control the bleeding so one part of your life doesn't screw up the other parts. Don't let a challenge at work disrupt your family life or vice versa.

11. Find purpose in the crisis ... the pony in the manure. People say everything happens for a reason. I'm not sure this is true. I think crap happens. It's our job, perhaps with God's help, to find the meaning and purpose in setbacks. Having purpose makes us more resilient. Viktor Frankl, a psychiatrist, Holocaust survivor and author of "Man's Search for Meaning," suggested that Despair = Suffering – Meaning. The more meaning we can find in our suffering, the more we can reduce our despair.

12. Consider how your situation could have been worse. Seems strange, right? This is from "Option B: Facing Adversity, Building Resilience and Finding Joy" by Sheryl Sandberg and Adam Grant. Sandberg emphasizes that what people should be looking for is a sense of gratitude, not a single jolt of happiness. As she grappled with losing her husband to heart failure as he was exercising on a treadmill, she eventually came to realize that her loss could have been worse. He could have died while he was driving their two children to school and she would have lost her entire family.

13. Practice the 13 skills of flourishing. Each of the 13 skills leads to greater resilience in the face of setbacks.

Reflections for the Second Half

- Have your previous setbacks and transitions followed the model presented?

- Are there setbacks you feel you've handled well? What helped you do so?

- How have setbacks shaped your life for the better?

- When have you experienced post-traumatic growth?

Quotes About Having Confidence in the Future

1. *"If you're walking through hell, keep walking."*
—WINSTON CHURCHILL

2. *"If you can meet with Triumph and Disaster*
And treat those two impostors just the same;
... And lose, and start again at your beginnings
... Yours is the Earth and everything that's in it."
—RUDYARD KIPLING

3. *"I choose to enjoy living the great mystery. The*
Tao that can be named is not the Tao."
—LAO-TZU

4. *"The Gods have two ways of blessing us. One is*
to grant our wishes, the other is to deny them."
—MODIFIED FROM OSCAR WILDE

5. *"Courage is not simply one of the virtues but*
the form of every virtue at the testing point, which
means at the point of highest reality."
—C.S. LEWIS

6. *"When one door of happiness closes, another opens;*
but often we look so long at the closed door that we do
not see the one which has been opened for us."
—HELEN KELLER

7. *"Difficulties are just things to overcome, after all."*
—SIR ERNEST SHACKLETON

8. *"Life is a storm, my young friend. You will bask in sunlight one moment, be shattered on the rocks the next. What makes you a man is what you do when that storm comes."*
—ALEXANDRE DUMAS

9. *"And now I'm glad I didn't know*
The way it all would end, the way it all would go
Our lives are better left to chance
I could have missed the pain
But I'd have had to miss the dance."
—GARTH BROOKS, "THE DANCE"

10. *"Sometimes we're the dog, sometimes the hydrant."*
—CHARLES SCHULZ

11. *"The most beautiful people we have known are those who have known defeat, known suffering, known struggle, known loss, and have found their way out of the depths. These persons have an appreciation, a sensitivity, and an understanding of life that fills them with compassion, gentleness, and a deep loving concern. Beautiful people do not just happen."*
—ELISABETH KÜBLER-ROSS

12. *"Forget about the perfect life, There is a crack, a crack in everything. That's how the light gets in."*
—LEONARD COHEN, "ANTHEM"
(MODIFIED BY DOUGLAS A. SMITH)

13. *"First there is the fall, and then we recover from the fall. Both are the mercy of God!"*
—LADY JULIAN OF NORWICH

14. *"Let me fall. The person I become will catch me."*
—UNKNOWN

15. *"I have taken thousands of people across [the river] and to all of them my river has been nothing but a hindrance on their journey. They have traveled for money and business, to weddings and on pilgrimages; the river has been in their way and the ferryman was there to take them quickly across the obstacle. However, amongst the thousands, there have been a few, four of five, to whom the river was not an obstacle. They have heard its voice and listened to it, and the river has become holy to them, as it has to me."*
—HERMANN HESSE, "SIDDHARTHA"

16. *"Life is just a trip until you lose your luggage, your way and your map; then you are on a journey."*
—DOUGLAS A. SMITH

17. "When we are no longer able to change our situation, we are challenged to change ourselves."

—VIKTOR FRANKL,
"MAN'S SEARCH FOR MEANING"

18. "I walked a mile with Pleasure;
She chatted all the way;
But left me none the wiser
For all she had to say.
I walked a mile with Sorrow;
And ne'er a word said she;
But, oh! The things I learned from her,
When Sorrow walked with me."

—ROBERT BROWNING HAMILTON,
"ALONG THE ROAD"

19. "I am looking for blessings not in disguise."

—UNKNOWN

20. "Yes, hope and despondency, pleasure and pain,
Are mingled together as in sunshine and rain."

—William Knox

FINDING JOY
IN THE PRESENT

Chapter 7

DOING NOW WHAT I AM DOING NOW

At any moment, the fully present mind may shatter time and burst into now.

—DAVID STEINDL-RAST

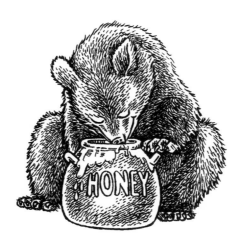

My mind has a mind of its own. It likes to jump from one topic to another and back again. It gets bored with the subject at hand almost regardless of what the subject is. Untrained, my mind can exhaust me, moving from the present, to the future, to the past again and again.

I also have some reactive qualities that are ingrained in well-traveled grooves that my mind enters in certain stressful situations. Most of these grooves do not serve me well. I am slowly calming and training my mind to be in the present, but I will admit I have much work to do.

Being in the present is one of the most difficult skills for most of us. Rather than being in the present, we are almost always distracted, feeling remorse or anger about the past or worrying about the future. Being able to learn from the past and prepare for the future are wonderful skills, skills unique to the human species. Unfortunately, most of us terribly misuse these skills, agonizing about things that happened half a lifetime ago and conjuring up all kinds of negative scenarios about how tomorrow will unfold. In doing this, we miss the opportunity to live with joy in the present. Happiness is found in the present, but we must be there to find it. Having our head be where our feet are, to be in the moment, is a wonderful skill. This skill of being in the present is made incredibly more difficult by the technology at our fingertips, which connects us to the world, but disconnects us from one another and from experiencing moments as we live them.

Anyone who plays sports has, at one time or another, "choked." I am now going to give you the definition of choking, so you will never choke again … as if it were that easy. Choking happens the second we step out of the present and into the past with anger or remorse, or we step into the future with fear and trepidation. In sports, this is called choking. In life, it is called unhappiness.

When I visit our vacation home in New York's Adirondack

Mountains, I often climb the mountain behind the house. As I look out over the lake I feel incredible peace. I think the reason I feel peace is because I am totally in the present. I don't need to change a thing; the moment is just perfect the way it is. I am 100% in the present.

Think back to moments when you were extremely happy and I'll bet they had this in common: They were moments when you were totally present, not worrying about the future or being angry or remorseful about the past. Like when your child was born, you had just graduated, or you were standing on a mountain gazing out at the horizon. These moments of being present are where happiness is found.

Alex Honnold is a world-renowned free climber. Free climbers climb without a rope, and Alex will tell you that his happiest times are when he is on the face of the cliff. It could be freezing cold, his fingers could be raw, he could be bruised and exhausted. Still, he would say it is among his happiest times. Why?

I think there are a couple of reasons why. One is Alex is using his unique talents to do something he thinks is important — staying alive. The other reason is that Alex is 100% in the present. He can't worry about what happened yesterday or last month. He can't think about the bills that haven't been paid or the meeting he has to go to tomorrow. Staying alive requires 100% of his focus on the face of the cliff. He is totally in the present and this brings him joy.

I used to think happiness was when I got promoted, went on vacation, or achieved some other life milestone. It was as if the time that I was traveling from A to B was just filler. I have come to realize that happiness is found in living not only in those special moments, but, more importantly, in the time traveling from A to B. It is in being present where I am, it is doing now what I am doing now. We don't have to wait for happiness; it is not for another place or another time, but for now, where we are.

How to Practice Being in the Present

Here are some ideas for doing now what I am doing now:

1. Stop multitasking. Multitasking is the enemy of happiness. Focus your attention on one thing at a time. You will find it much more enjoyable and your work will improve significantly. This includes trying to read the paper, watch TV, read an email, etc., while you talk to your spouse or kids or co-workers.

2. Practice "thresholds." Several years ago, I worked with a personal coach who noticed my tendency to always be doing several things at once, or "multitasking." She taught me the skill of "thresholds." Here is how it works: Every time we pass through a doorway we should think of the doorway as a threshold. Once through the threshold, we should concentrate on what is on that side of the threshold, that side of the doorway. When you drive home at night and pass from the garage door into the house, think of that garage doorway as a threshold and concentrate on what is happening in the home, not the office, not the bad traffic, and not the guy who cut you off on your way home.

When I told the personal coach I often need to do work at home, she said, "Use the same tool. If you have an office at home or a room you work in, pass through that doorway. Your family will know you need to be working." She went on to say, "What I don't want you to do is sit in front of the TV, read the paper, speak to your kids or wife, and check your cell phone for messages. I want you to do one thing at a time." "Thresholds" are a great tool to help you be present where you are.

3. The one minute pause. Here is a simple tool to bring you into the present. Several times a day, stop whatever you are doing and take a pause. Breathe in slowly and imagine that you are breathing in whatever you desire — peace, calmness, joy, love, insight. Then slowly exhale, imagining that you are releasing whatever you want to release — stress, tension, worry, anger. Do this for four or five deep breaths. There are both physiological and psychological reasons this works. Physiologically, slowing your breath engages your parasympathetic nervous system through your vagus nerve. This tells your body that everything is OK and reduces heart rate and blood pressure, basically calming you down. From a psychological perspective, focusing on your breath brings you into the present, enabling you to release anger or remorse about the past and trepidation about the future. If you suffer from high blood pressure, this is a particularly good exercise.

4. Meditation. Meditation is a key to mindfulness. Meditation helps us directly experience the present without judgment. Since meditation is also a key to spirituality we will cover this skill in more detail in the next chapter.

Reflections for the Second Half

- How much time do you spend being in the present each day?

- Would you like to spend more time being in the present? If so, what prevents you from doing so?

- If you would like to spend more time in the present, what two or three actions could you take to do so?

Quotes About Doing Now What I Am Doing Now

1. "Eternal life is given to those who live in the present."

—LUDWIG WITTGENSTEIN

2. "At any moment, the fully present mind may shatter time and burst into now."

—DAVID STEINDL-RAST

3. "Yesterday is ashes, tomorrow wood. Only today the fire burns brightly."

—OLD ESKIMO PROVERB

4. "We all need a dog tag that says, 'Stay. Sit. Heal.'"

—PEMA CHÖDRÖN

5. "To be absolutely nothing, is to be everything."

—JAMES W. DOUGLASS

6. "To meet everything and everyone through stillness instead of mental noise is the greatest gift you can offer to the universe."

—ECKHART TOLLE

7. *"Happiness is not in another place, but in this place ... not another hour, but this hour."*
                    —WALT WHITMAN, "LEAVES OF GRASS"

8. *"Choking happens the second we step out of the present and into the past with anger or remorse, or we step into the future with fear and trepidation. In sports, this is called choking. In life, it is called unhappiness."*
                    —DOUGLAS A. SMITH

Chapter 8

Honoring Mind, Body & Spirit

To whom and to what do you give access to your mind, your body and your spirit?

—DENNIS BLAND

We live with greater joy when we care for our entire selves — our mind, body and spirit. Taking care of ourselves is not selfish. If we want to be of help to others, the first thing we must do is take care of ourselves. Honoring our mind, body and spirit is key to flourishing — and this self-care takes on even greater importance as we age.

My friend Dennis Bland leads the Center for Leadership Development, or CLD, in Indianapolis. The CLD is dedicated to enabling inner-city black youths to become successful adults. The organization runs courses in the evening and on weekends for some 2,500 students aged 7 to 22.

Dennis always asks this question of program participants: "To whom and to what do you give access to your mind, your body and your spirit?" It's a question we need to ask ourselves repeatedly. If we are not happy with the answer, we need to make changes.

Let's start with our bodies. The body is the source of our energy and energy is what enables us to move, work and play. To perform optimally, our bodies need healthy food, good sleep and regular exercise. When we neglect or abuse our bodies, it is at our peril. Many of us reach the end of the day and wonder why we are exhausted. The solution may be as simple as taking better care of our bodies.

If you leave what you eat and drink to the food and beverage companies, you will be very disappointed with the results. The food companies know that fat and sugar, especially in combination, light up the pleasure centers of our brains. The more fat and sugar they use, the more addictive their product becomes. They also know if they make it really easy to chew (think chicken nuggets), add contrasting flavors (spicy chicken nuggets with cool ranch sauce) and give us bigger portions (all you can eat), we will be in hog heaven.

Today, the average American weighs 28 pounds more than in 1960, and more than 35% of us are obese. In 1960, only 10% of us were obese. It doesn't have to be this way. In Japan, just 3.5% of the population is obese. It's estimated that 50% of us will be obese in 2040 if we don't change our habits.

We don't have to be model thin or weigh what we did in college, but being significantly overweight bears a heavy burden on our hearts and our joints, is associated with several forms of cancer and is a leading cause of diabetes. It can hurt our self-image, our self-esteem. Combine being overweight with a sedentary lifestyle and you are likely drastically reducing the quality and length of life.

Changing habits takes time, with careful consideration for how to become more active and lose weight. When it comes to exercise, the American Heart Association recommends at least 30 minutes of vigorous activity five days a week. Ideally, this exercise would include both aerobic activity, free weights and stretching to foster flexibility. If you have been inactive, it would be best to seek medical advice before starting an exercise routine, but it's never too late to start moving.

Sleep is also important. Many of us tend to be sleep warriors, priding ourselves on how little sleep we need. But lack of sleep negatively impacts us physically, intellectually and emotionally. Experts recommend seven to eight hours of sleep each night on a regular schedule, meaning we go to bed and rise at approximately the same time each day. In this regard, "early to bed and early to rise" is great advice for making us more productive and happier.

Now think about your mind. Who and what has access to it? What do you read? Watch on TV? Who do you socialize with? What websites do you visit? The goal is to have a healthy, informed and peaceful mind. In the second half of life maintaining our intellectual curiosity, reading, staying informed and remaining mentally agile takes on increased importance.

A note regarding our 24-hour "news" channels: Media outlets on both the left and the right work hard to get us angry over what the "other side" is up to. Being consistently angry weighs heavily on our ability to flourish. Negative emotions drain our energy, while positive emotions ignite energy. Find media outlets that lift your spirits. This is particularly important in the hour or so before you go to bed.

Finally, let's consider honoring our spirit. Spirituality is a journey to one's inner self to discover who we were intended to be. In a world of chaos, we need a sense of grounding that can only be found within. We live so much of our lives looking outside ourselves for solutions to our problems, for our happiness and for our sense of self. Most of us have a self-worth chasm that at times is huge. The world would have us try to fill this chasm with trinkets ... a new BMW, a new pair of shoes, a promotion at work, a facelift. After a quick hit of "happiness," these things just leave us feeling emptier.

What we seek is not outside ourselves, but inside ourselves. Spirituality is a journey to find our inner sacred self. It is about stopping, reflecting and using our inner voice to put the disparate pieces of our life together in some form of a harmonious, peaceful, meaningful, grounded whole. If we believe in God or a larger presence, it is a journey to be at one with that presence. Whatever we believe, we won't make this journey without reflection or silence ... and silence is so hard to achieve in our perpetually connected world.

We live in a world increasingly devoid of spirituality. Everything is immediate and transactional. We don't have time for reflection, introspection, or to develop a deeper sense of character — an understanding of what is kind or unkind, just or unjust, loving or unloving. More often, we occupy our time with nonsubstantive forms of communication and "electronic relationships" through our phones and computers. This lack of spirituality makes it more difficult to deal with traumatic events, or a future that doesn't turn out as we hoped. To better cope, we need a deeper sense of who we are.

How to Practice Honoring Our Mind, Body & Spirit

1. PIES. Think about your Physical, Intellectual, Emotional and Spiritual needs and determine how you can better meet these needs. You cannot take care of or help others unless you take care of yourself. Be sure you are recognizing the importance of caring for yourself.

2. Silence. Make time for silence each day. Carve out a half hour each day for silence. Silence offers the opportunity to escape the chaotic, unreal, materialistic world we live in. In welcoming silence, we shut out advertising, Facebook, television, YouTube and many other external commercial channels and invite the opportunity to think and examine our emotions. Through prayer, meditation and reflection — all of which require silence — we can begin to center ourselves and increasingly think, feel and act in a more truthful, positive and joyful manner.

3. Journaling. Taking time to capture in writing your thoughts, your answers to life's deeper questions, can illuminate and aid your spiritual journey.

4. Service. Using your talents to benefit others can increase your sense of self-worth and deepen the meaning and gratitude you feel. Helping others helps us see how blessed we are.

5. Meditate. This may be the most powerful of the tools we share. Meditation has the power to transform our lives in many ways. It is the key to mindfulness, the ability to directly experience the present without judgment. Before we even think about how to meditate, let me take you through some of the benefits of meditation. Even Harvard Business Review — a business-focused publication you might not expect to embrace such a practice — recognizes the importance of meditation. Researchers have found that meditation:

- Builds resilience ("grit") and the ability to perform well under stress;

- Increases our emotional intelligence and our ability to regulate our emotions;

- Enhances creativity and enables us to have more "eureka" moments;

- Improves relationships, making us kinder and more compassionate; and

- Enables us to better focus and avoid distractions.

*Source: Harvard Business Review, "How Meditation Benefits CEOs," December 2015.

Meditation helps us better understand our minds. It helps us weed out the babble that too often dictates how we think and feel.

Here are some fundamentals about meditation that can help you get started if you are new to the concept:

- Try sitting quietly for just a few minutes each day. It

is best to do this first thing in the morning to set the tone for your day. If morning doesn't work for you, pick another time, but try to allocate the same time each day. You may wonder, "What am I supposed to do while I am doing this?" Don't even consider this, just try to do nothing. After a few days, see if you can lengthen the amount of time you sit quietly.

- After doing this for a week or so, start concentrating on your breath. Focus your attention on the space just beyond your nose, where your breath enters and leaves your body. It might help to count as you breathe in and again as you breathe out. Each time your mind wanders from your breath, gently bring it back to your breath. Think of such wandering as just another opportunity to practice bringing your mind back to where you want to focus. Be compassionate with yourself.

- As you progress in your ability to stay focused, you might try doing a body scan. Start at your feet and move upward, or start at your head and move downward. Think about how each area of your body feels. If you find discomfort, see if you can wiggle it out by focusing on it and releasing it.

- Gradually lengthen the time you sit quietly, adding a few minutes each day, until you reach 20 minutes.

- You can try guided meditation, if you think it would be helpful. I have "monkey brain," my mind likes to jump around from one thing to another even during meditation. Guided meditation helps me stay focused. There are many applications to help you meditate available in your app store, like Headspace,

Calm, Joy, etc.

- Reflect on how you feel after you meditate. Do you feel more peaceful? Do you begin to have greater awareness and mastery of your thoughts? Do you feel more centered, less stressed? If so, keep up the practice. Consider finding a community or guide to improve your skills.

A Harvard study found those who meditate 20 minutes or more a day actually rewire their brains for greater serenity and mastery of their emotions.

Reflections for the Second Half

- Which of the following — mind, body or spirit — could you benefit by honoring better?

- What steps would you like to commit to taking to do so?

Quotes About Honoring Mind, Body & Spirit

1. *"Wholeness is not achieved by cutting off a portion of one's being, but by integration of the contraries."*

—CARL JUNG

2. *"Let's build wellness rather than treating disease."*

—BRUCE DAGGY

3. *"Self-care is so important. When you take time to replenish your spirit, it allows you to serve others from the overflow. You cannot serve from an empty vessel."*

—ELEANOR BROWN

4. *"Your mind, emotions and body are instruments and the way you align and tune them determines how well you play life."*

—HARBHAJAN SINGH YOGI

5. *"A sound mind in a sound body is a short but full description of a happy state in this world."*

—JOHN LOCKE

6. *"Spirituality is about looking beyond the surface of things. It opens you to explore and connect more deeply with what brings meaning, value and purpose to your life. Along the way, you'll cultivate a more meaningful view of yourself in relation to the world."*

—CANYON RANCH

7. *"Spirituality ignites passion, which leads to exploration of new and exciting depths of imagination and experience. Following your deepest yearning to establish a connection with spirit, you come home to your truest self."*

—CANYON RANCH

8. *"To whom and to what do you give access to your mind, your body and your spirit?"*

—DENNIS BLAND

9. *"Spiritual connections help you cope with life's adversities, leading to reduced stress and anxiety, better health habits, stronger support systems, and a more optimistic and resilient nature."*

—MEL ZUCKERMAN

Chapter 9

ALTRUISM / KINDNESS

It is one of the most beautiful compensations of this life that no man can sincerely try to help another without helping himself.

—RALPH WALDO EMERSON

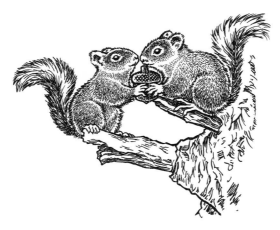

Martin Seligman often tells a story of finding happiness on a trip to the post office to buy one-cent stamps. Before Forever Stamps existed, people had to buy one-cent stamps each time the postal rate increased to round up the value of the stamps they already had. One time Seligman arrived at the post office to buy one-cent stamps, there was a long line snaking out the door. After waiting a half hour, he arrived at the counter. Instead of buying the 20 stamps, or 20¢ worth, he needed, he bought 2,000 stamps, or $20 worth. He then turned around to the assembled line and said, "One-cent stamps! Who needs them?" He proceeded to walk up to each person, saying, "How many do you need?" and gave them what they asked for. When he left, everyone in line gave him a standing ovation. He says it was one of the happiest days of his life.

Practicing kindness is key to flourishing. This is not about doing one or two acts of kindness a day. It is about kindness as a way of life.

Kindness or altruism not only does good, it feels good.

We are wired to be kind and to help one another. This could be why we have survived as a species in a dangerous world with predators far stronger than we humans. Kindness, cooperation and care for one another are in our genes.

Kindness actually lights up the pleasure centers of our brains. Positive psychologists conducted a study where they gave individuals $20. Half the group was told to go out and buy something nice for themselves. The other half was told to go buy something nice for a friend or someone in need. Several days later, the psychologists measured each group's level of happiness. Those who bought a gift for someone else were measurably happier. Scientists have found that performing an act of kindness produces the single most reliable momentary increase in well-being of any exercise they have tested.

People in business settings often seem to think kindness has little to do with work. On the contrary, effective teamwork and leadership require it. Start with the assumption that leadership is given, not grabbed. Power and influence are given to the most successful leaders by the people who follow them. People give power to those who act in the collective best interest. When leaders are motivated by self-interest and not the best interest of others, followers eventually turn away or undermine their power.

Numerous studies across a broad range of arenas, including manufacturing plants, banks, schools and hospitals, found successful leaders generally act in five ways. These social tendencies have been named the "Big Five":

- **Enthusiasm:** They reach out to others.

- **Focus:** They focus on shared goals.

- **Kindness:** They cooperate, share, care about others.

- **Calmness:** They instill calm, perspective ... they are the eye of the storm.

- **Openness:** They are open to others' ideas, feelings, needs.*

*Source: "The Power Paradox: How We Gain and Lose Influence," by Dacher Keltner

The conclusion I've come to is that "being altruistic/kind" leads not only to happiness but more effective leadership and better organization performance. Kindness is critical to flourishing for individuals and enterprises. Incivility and lack of kindness cost companies billions of dollars each year. Just ask United Airlines how much incivility cost them after a passenger was violently dragged off one of their planes to make room for a United Airlines employee. The stock market value of the airline dropped by more than $1 billion the next day.

We are instinctively drawn to certain people more than others. These people are generally more charismatic, and a key part of charisma is kindness. Olivia Fox Cabane, author of "The Charisma Myth: How Anyone Can Master the Art and Science of Personal Magnetism," suggests there are three qualities that comprise charisma. The first is presence, which involves residing in the moment. When charismatic people are with you, they give you their full attention. They make you feel valued. The second is power. Charismatic people are comfortable with themselves and their position of authority. The last is warmth. Cabane describes this as "a certain kind of vibe that signals kindness and acceptance."

David Brooks considers "being altruistic/kind" the route to "moral joy," the highest state of motivation humans can achieve. He wrote about his theory in a Sept. 23, 2017, editorial in the New York Times titled "When Life Asks for Everything."

He compared two models of motivational theory, looking first at Maslow's hierarchy of needs. Maslow believes we must meet our physiological needs before we can move onto others. Once we fulfill our physiological needs, we can move on to safety, then love/belonging, self-esteem and, finally, self-actualization. For Maslow, the pinnacle of existence is self-actualization.

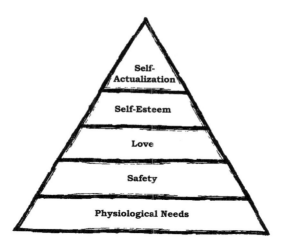

Brooks prefers another model he calls "Four Kinds of Happiness." At the base is material pleasure, like having food, clothing and shelter. Next is achievement, or the pleasure derived from earned recognized success. This is followed by generativity, or the pleasure derived from giving back to others. At the top is what he calls "moral joy." He describes moral joy as "the glowing satisfaction we get when we have surrendered ourselves to some noble cause or unconditional love."

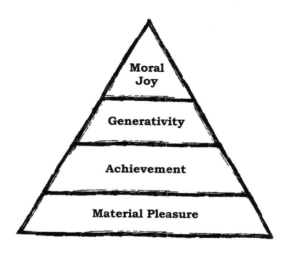

The difference between these two models is that Maslow's moves from the collective and relational to the self. While Brooks' model moves from the individual, or self, to the relational and finally the collective. I think his model is enlightening. The happiest among us live not in an independent world, but in an interdependent world, where we are engaged in, even surrendered to, helping others. Kindness leads to moral joy.

One final point on kindness: Often when we see, hear or read about an unexpected act of kindness, we have a feeling of benevolence ourselves. There is an explanation for this sensation. Psychologists call it "elevation." Thomas Jefferson was one of the first people to write about elevation: "When an act of charity or of gratitude is presented to our sight or imagination, we are deeply impressed with its beauty and feel a strong desire within ourselves of doing charitable and grateful acts also. It can elevate our bodies and mind, opening our chest and hearts." Kindness begets kindness.

How to Practice Altruism/Kindness

1. Be kind to everyone, including yourself. You won't be kind to others if you are not kind to yourself. As they say when you fly, "Put your own oxygen mask on first before you try to help others." Before most every action you take, ask yourself, "Is this kind?" If it isn't, consider a different action.

2. Be interested. Everyone wants to be interesting, but it starts with being interested. Showing someone you are interested in what they are doing or saying is an act of kindness.

3. Be patient and listen. Patience is waiting without fear. When someone is speaking, don't interrupt them or complete their sentences. Have the patience to hear them out. Give them your undivided attention, even if they drone on. Accept that people have different styles of communicating. (More on this later in the Cherishing Relationships chapter.)

5. Give up gossip. Do not spread negative stories about others. Find the good and focus on that.

Reflections for the Second Half

- What causes do you feel most passionate about?

- Are there people in your life who seek you out for counsel and help? Could you give them more attention, benefiting you both?

- What talents and resources do you have that might be more fully utilized to improve this world?

Quotes About Altruism/Kindness

1. *"It is one of the most beautiful compensations of this life that no man can sincerely try to help another without helping himself."*
                                    —RALPH WALDO EMERSON

2. *"The most important factor in the survival of Homo sapiens is our social nature, our ability to love one another and work together."*
                                    —ELLEN BERSCHEID

3. *"The true meaning of life is to plant trees under whose shade you do not expect to sit."*
                                    —NELSON HENDERSON

4. *"A tribe including many members who ... were always ready to aid one another to sacrifice themselves for the common good; this would be natural selection."*
                                    —CHARLES DARWIN

5. *"Giving is the greatest form of appreciation because it is appreciation in action. It is not philosophy, it is an experience. The experience takes you outside yourself and pulls you away from your problems, fears and self-involvement."*
                                    —DAN BAKER

6. *"Altruism has been called the great paradox. When you give something to someone else, you're the one who feels best. Giving is getting. Studies show that happy people are altruistic, and that altruistic people are happy."*

—DAN BAKER

7. *"Survival of the kindest may be just as fitting a description of our origins as survival of the fittest."*

—DACHER KELTNER

8. *"Ubuntu"* (What happens to others, happens to me.)

—SOUTH AFRICAN WORD

9. *"The cost of my survival must have been hundreds of millions of dollars. All to save one dorky botanist. Why bother? ... because every human being has a basic instinct to help each other out. This is so fundamentally human that it's found in every culture without exception."*

—ANDY WEIR, "THE MARTIAN"

10. *"The secret to inner peace and lasting happiness is kindness. Not random acts, but kindness as a way of life."*

—WAYNE DYER

Chapter 10

THINKING WITH ABUNDANCE

In our research, we asked people whom they compete against. The unhappiest went on and on while the happiest didn't know what we were talking about.

—SONJA LYUBOMIRSKY

I will admit that I am a very competitive person. Many of us view that as a strength, and for most of my life, so did I. In my late thirties I took a Life Style Inventory test. Many of you may have taken such a test. It measures 12 behavioral styles, such as being humanistic, perfectionistic, self-actualizing and competitive. My results came back and I was off the charts on being competitive. As I began to gloat and suggest, "Well, I was a bit of an athlete in college," the psychologist reviewing the results stopped me mid-sentence, saying, "Doug, I want you to know this is not a positive trait." My response and belief for the next number of years was, "That is ridiculous. Of course, being competitive is a positive trait. It's what makes me successful; it drives me each day to be more successful."

I am sure several of you are nodding your heads. My psychologist proceeded to share with me the characteristics of someone who is highly competitive. His description fit me perfectly. Here is what he said, "Those who are highly competitive seek self-worth through competing and comparing themselves to others. They seek self-esteem through being better than others. Being highly competitive is not a predictor of success in business or in sports. Rather those who are less competitive and focus more on performance excellence do better in most of life's domains. Highly competitive people have a deep-seated need for recognition and praise, have an extreme fear of failure and tend to be overly aggressive."

My guess is that most of you reading this are still not buying the idea that being highly competitive is not a virtue. Probably because most of you think that being competitive is what makes or made you successful. Most likely, being competitive played a part. But as the Life Style Inventory finding above indicates, we pay a price for being highly competitive and, importantly, there may be a more effective way to behave that can lead to even greater success. If you would, suspend your judgment for just a little while longer.

Comparison is the Thief of Joy

Competition is about scarcity. Competition is fueled by believing the world only has so much to offer — if someone else gets something, it means there is less for me. The analogy would be considering the world as a pie; if someone else gets a piece, then there is that much less to go around. Abundance is the opposite. Basically, it's believing the world is abundant and there is plenty of pie for everyone. If someone gets a piece, well, the pie just gets that much bigger.

I teach at Canyon Ranch. If you asked me 10 years ago what my objective was, I would have answered, "To be the best teacher at Canyon Ranch." Maybe you think this is a good objective. I have come to believe that it is not. In fact, that objective does not serve me, the guests at Canyon Ranch or Canyon Ranch very well. A better objective for me is, "To help people, to the best of my ability, understand and practice the skills that lead to a meaningful, accomplished, joyful life ... that lead to flourishing."

My objective 10 years ago is fueled by competition, it is about scarcity. It is driven by fear and my ego, and it is all about ME. And yes, it will get me to work hard. But It prevents me from sharing information with other teachers at Canyon Ranch because they might prevent me from reaching my goal of being the best. It also puts the achievement of my objective, to a certain degree, in someone else's hands.

The second objective is not about ego, but about conscience. It is "other" inspired in that it is directed not at myself, but the people I teach. The second objective encourages me to share with and learn from other instructors at Canyon Ranch. It has nothing to do with competition. It is about abundance, about cooperation, about love. It will inspire me more than the first objective to be a better teacher. The second objective benefits the guests at Canyon Ranch, the other teachers and me. Cooperation beats out competition in most every endeavor.

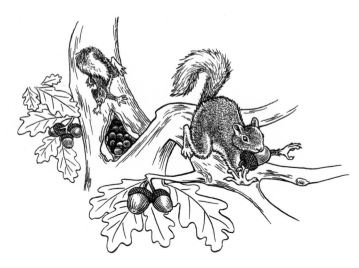

Being less competitive doesn't mean we have to give up our edge. If we live with abundance, we will stand out from the crowd because so few of us are inspired by love. I think this was the lesson I should have taken away from my Life Style Inventory test 30 years ago, but didn't. It took me the past 20 years to fully grasp this. I am glad I better understand it today, even if I still struggle with practicing abundance consistently.

This lesson holds for almost every species. I am currently reading a book by Peter Wohlleben titled "The Hidden Life of Trees." It is excellent. His primary contention is that trees cooperate and communicate with one another constantly, and without this cooperation, we would have no trees:

"Trees in the forest care for one another, sometimes even going so far as to nourish a stump of a felled tree for centuries after it has been cut down by feeding it sugars and other nutrients, and so keeping it alive. A tree's most important means of staying connected to other trees is a 'wood wide web' of soil fungi that connects vegetation in an intimate network that allows sharing an enormous amount of information and goods. The reason they share food and communicate is that they need each other. It takes a forest to create a microclimate suitable for tree growth and sustenance."

Just as trees need each other, we need each other. I believe that if we can view the world with abundance, if we can be motivated by cooperation and not competition, by conscience rather than ego, and if we are inspired by love rather than driven by fear, we will be more successful and live with greater joy ... we will flourish.

Are you competitive? Here are a couple of situations that will help you determine whether you are or not:

1. You come to a stoplight and a car pulls up next to you. They seem to want to go faster than you. The road 200 yards ahead narrows to one lane. You were at the light first. What do you do when the light changes? If you try to beat them, you are being competitive and thinking with scarcity.

2. Your best friend just got something you would like to have — a new BMW, a promotion, a new second home. You say to them, "Congratulations. I am so happy for you." But how do you really feel? If you feel anything but joy for the person, you are thinking with scarcity.

I have to admit it's difficult to get beyond a scarcity state of mind. When someone else gets something I would desperately like to have, it still sometimes feels as if the desired thing was heading right for me and the other person reached up and grabbed it before I could. Abundance enables us to experience "sympathetic joy," where we actually feel joy in witnessing another's joy. I am working to experience more of this.

How to Practice Abundance

1. Stop comparing yourself to others. Other people's success has little to do with your success. Think of the world as unlimited in terms of opportunity. Think of your success or objectives as absolutes, versus measuring yourself relative to others. Seek to be the best you can be and help others do the same.

2. Establish objectives that are other-centered, rather than setting goals of being better than others. Measure progress by how well you meet these other-centered objectives and how much you improve; no one else should figure into the equation.

3. Take joy in other people's accomplishments. When a friend or colleague is successful, find a way to feel joy rather than envy. Realize it is an abundant world.

Reflections for the Second Half

- Do you consider yourself a highly competitive person? Do you view this as a strength?

- If you think it would be better to focus more on cooperation than competition, how might you make this shift?

Quotes About Abundance

1. *"Every time a friend of mine succeeds, I die a little."*
—GORE VIDAL

2. *"The moment we begin to consider our worth by comparing ourselves to others, we are into scarcity thinking. When we compare ourselves to others, every benefit that accrues to them, by definition, diminishes us. Abundant thinkers do not seek their worth in comparison to others."*
—DACHER KELTNER

3. *"One of the sanest, surest and most generous joys of life comes from being happy over the good fortune of others."*
—ARCHIBALD RUTLEDGE

4. *"In our research, we asked people whom they compete against. The unhappiest went on and on while the happiest didn't know what we were talking about."*
—SONJA LYUBOMIRSKY

5. *"Mature people are not 'either-or' thinkers, but they bathe in the ocean of 'both-and.'"*
—RICHARD ROHR

6. *"...People who come out ahead in competitive situations focus on performance excellence or the process of doing well, rather than on the end result of winning."*

      —LIFE STYLE INVENTORY TEST

7. *"There is nothing noble in being superior to your fellow man; true nobility is being superior to your former self."*

      —ERNEST HEMINGWAY

Chapter 11

MASTERING OUR STORIES

Sometimes the most important conversations we have are the ones we have with ourselves.
—JIM LOEHR

Each of us has a voice inside our heads. If right now you are saying to yourself, "I don't have a voice inside my head," that is the voice I am talking about. The voice starts talking when you first wake up and continues all day long. It can even talk long after you have gone to bed and wish you were asleep.

Most of us aren't even aware of this roommate we carry with us. Once we realize we have this voice, most of us think that the voice is ours. It is not. We are the one listening, not the one talking. And we can choose whether or not to listen to this voice. This realization has tremendous power. The stories we tell ourselves shape our lives. In fact, we become the stories we tell ourselves.

Most of us think that the world works like this: We experience some event, we have an emotional response that makes us feel a particular way and then we respond.

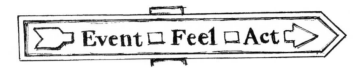

Actually, it's not quite that simple. Between "event" and "feel" there is something very important you create somewhere in your mind that determines how you feel and act. What happens in between the event and how we feel is that we tell ourselves a story. We mess with the data and put a particular spin around it and it is this story, rather than the event, that we respond to. We tell ourselves a story about everything that happens to us ... no exceptions.

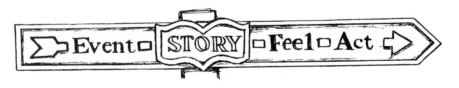

The other day, my wife Phyllis was driving and I was sitting in the passenger seat. We were in a long line of traffic for an exit. Some guy pulls ahead of everyone and cuts in toward the front of the line. I mutter to myself, "What a jerk!" Phyllis has no reaction. So, I said, "Doesn't that bother you? Look at that jerk — he thinks the rules don't apply to him. He doesn't care about anyone else!"

She looked over at me and said: "How do you know that? Maybe he is running to the hospital because his wife is having a baby. Maybe his boss told him if he is late to the meeting today he is fired. Maybe he is trying to catch a flight." Now I think my story might have been more accurate than Phyllis's in this particular situation, but the point I want to make is that it is the story we tell ourselves that determines our response, not the event itself.

So how do we tell ourselves these stories? Not so kindly it turns out.

Do you know the country song "Jukebox in My Mind"? Well, guess what? The jukebox usually is playing terrible songs. For most of us, the voice inside our heads is the voice of fear and shouts things about others we would never say out loud and tells us things about ourselves we would never let someone else say. Dan Harris of ABC News has written a book titled "10% Happier." He originally wanted to title it "The Voice Inside My Head is an Asshole." I know how he feels.

Here's the point: Master the stories you tell yourself and you become master of your life. Be a servant to the voice and you'll always be at the mercy of a fearful child.

We often use the stories we tell ourselves to justify not doing something we should be doing or to keep doing something we shouldn't. Here's an example of a story I told myself for years that kept me from changing: "I have a short temper because my Dad had a short temper." Translation: "Hey, it's not my fault I get angry, it's my Dad's fault. There is nothing I can do about it." If I keep telling myself that story, I will always have a short temper.

As Srikumar Rao puts it, "Our lives are hemmed in by things we know to be true ... that aren't." Our stories define and confine us.

I used to tell myself this story: "I am not good with names." Guess what? As long as I told myself that story I wasn't good with names. I gave up that story and changed it to: "There is no reason I can't be good with names." Now I concentrate when I meet people. Guess what? Now I do pretty well with people's names.

We tell ourselves stories about work, family, relatives, friends, health, happiness, money, what we can do, what we can't do, about the boss, about our co-workers, about our kids, our parents ... you get the idea. We tell ourselves stories about everything and everyone.

Some stories we tell ourselves once and they make little difference in our lives. My "I am not good with names" story did not have that big an impact on my life. Some stories we tell ourselves for a few weeks. Some we tell ourselves for a lifetime and they shape the very character of our existence.

The stories we tell ourselves are the only reality we know. We all tell some dysfunctional stories. But a preponderance of dysfunctional stories leads to a dysfunctional life. Recognizing the stories that don't serve us well is a first step in mastering our stories. When you change your stories, you change your life.

Here are some stories that maybe, just maybe, you are telling yourself:

- My work prevents me from exercising.

- No one in my position is happy.

- I don't have time to eat well.

- I will never forgive my mother ... brother ... wife/husband ... son/daughter ... friend.

- I am overweight because my parents were overweight.

- Fear of failure makes me successful ... insecurity is the price I pay for security.

- I will start saving when I get my next promotion.

- I will start spending more time with my family when I get my next promotion.

- I will be happy when the kids leave home ... and then ... I will be happy when the kids come home.

- I will be happy when my spouse treats me better.

And here are two different stories that lead to very different outcomes:

- Both my parents were alcoholics. Of course, I have an alcohol problem. What do you expect?

- Both my parents were alcoholics. Of course, I don't drink. What do you expect?

I want to take this concept of story a little deeper. I recently read "A Million Miles in a Thousand Years" by Donald Miller. Here is his opening sentence: "Nobody cries at the end of a movie [story] about a guy who wants to buy a Volvo." He goes on to write that the reason they don't cry is because it's not a good story. If what we do with our lives won't make a good story, it won't make a good life either. He defines a good story as, "A character who wants something and overcomes conflict to get it." He goes on to describe an epic story as, "A character who wants something that is very difficult such that his/ her very life may even be in jeopardy and what he/she wants is for the sake of someone else ... it is sacrificial."

So here are the questions I think Miller is subtly challenging us to ask ourselves: What is our life story? Does our life story make a good story? A good life? Is our life story sacrificial? Stories that lean toward being epic are ones founded on a meaningful purpose that benefits our world ... and finding that purpose is the focus of our next chapter.

As performance psychologist Jim Loehr says, "Your life is your story. Your story is your life."

How to Practice Mastering Our Stories

- **First, just listen to your voice for a couple of days.** Most of us don't even know we have this voice, though we have been listening to it all our lives.

- **Then ask yourself if the voice is helpful.** What is its tone — harsh, helpful, mean-spirited, kind? Is it even my voice or is it someone else's, like my Mom or Dad's? Will it get me where I want to go and help me be the person I want to be? If not, take the next two steps.

- **Give the voice a name.** I call mine Rex because it is a voice of fear originating in the most primitive parts of my brain ... the reptilian brain.

- **Change the story.** Now when the voice speaks, recognize it for what it is. The voice never goes away, but if it isn't helpful, you don't have to listen to it. The more you ignore it, the quieter it gets. You can then begin to change the story you tell yourself. You will eventually become the master of your inner voice as opposed to its servant.

Reflections for the Second Half

- How have the stories you tell yourself shaped your life?

- What specific stories would you like to change?

- What kind of story will your life make? Will it be a good story? Does the story of the second half move in the direction of being epic?

Quotes About Mastering Our Stories

1. *"The mind is a wonderful servant, but a terrible master."*

—UNKNOWN

2. *"Your life is your story. Your story is your life."*
—JIM LOEHR

3. *"Our lives are hemmed in by things we know to be true ... that aren't."*
—SRIKUMAR RAO

4. *"If an idiot told you the same story for a year, you would end by believing it."*
—HORACE MANN

5. *"More important than the facts of our life experiences are the stories we inevitably tell ourselves about these facts."*
—DOUGLAS A. SMITH

6. *"Sometimes the most important conversations we have are the ones we have with ourselves."*
—JIM LOEHR

7. *"Between stimulus and response there is a space. In that space is our power to choose our response. In our response lies our growth and freedom."*

—VIKTOR FRANKL

8. *"Often we don't need new facts, we need new stories."*

—JIM LOEHR

9. *"Among all the things we don't control, we do have control over our stories. Individual responsibility is contained in the act of selecting and constantly revising the master narrative we tell about ourselves. The most important power we have is the power to help select the lens through which we see reality."*

—DAVID BROOKS

Chapter 12

FINDING PURPOSE

To be in hell is to drift; to be in heaven is to steer.
—GEORGE BERNARD SHAW

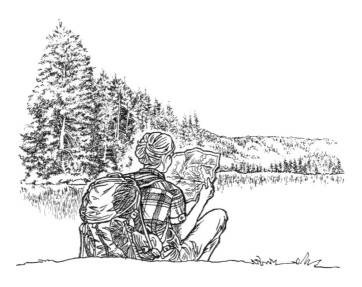

At the foundation of the ability to flourish in life are two fundamental skills: purpose and relationships. Figure these two lodestars out — that is, identify and passionately pursue meaningful purpose(s) and have healthy, enduring relationships — and your chances of living a flourishing life are enhanced many times over. In this chapter, we will deal with purpose and in the next relationships.

Remember the movie "Cast Away"? It revolves around a FedEx employee named Chuck Noland, played by Tom Hanks, who is marooned for nearly five years on a South Pacific island. The movie has several symbolic props important to our hero's survival over the years he is marooned. There are two specific props — a FedEx box and a soccer ball — we'll discuss in this and the following chapter.

First, let's look at the FedEx box. During Noland's first few days on the island, several FedEx packages wash up on the beach. Noland proceeds to open the boxes, finding uses for most of the items: an ice skate becomes an ax, a ballet tutu becomes a fishing net, etc. When he gets to the last package, he starts to open it, stops, and sets it aside. He leaves it unopened. When he finally leaves the island, he takes the unopened package with him.

Why would he do this? I think it's because the package gives Noland purpose. Perhaps he was thinking something like this: "I am a FedEx employee. Somehow I am going to get off this damn island and deliver this package." And he does deliver it once he returns. When he drops off the package, no one is home and he leaves this note with the box: "This package saved my life."

Much of what saves us all from lives of quiet desperation is purpose. Our souls need purpose as much as our bodies need food.

In the book "Pathfinders," author Gail Sheehy met with hundreds of people she thought were living joyful, meaningful, accomplished lives ... people who were flourishing. She concluded they all possessed 10 specific qualities. No. 1 was: "My life has meaning and purpose." Purpose is key to flourishing.

The 13 skills we cover in this book are all essential to each of the 10 attributes Sheehy identifies, so I am listing all the attributes here:

- My life has meaning and purpose.

- I have experienced one or more important transitions in my adult years, and I have handled these in an unusual, personal or creative way.

- I rarely feel cheated or disappointed by life.

- I have attained several of the long-term goals that are important to me.

- I am pleased with my personal growth and development.

- I am in love; my partner and I love mutually.

- I have many friends.

- I am a cheerful person.

- I am not thin-skinned or sensitive to criticism.

- I have no major fears.

Others have also underscored the importance of purpose in our lives. Prime among them is Viktor Frankl. A noted Austrian psychologist in the 1940s, Frankl was imprisoned in a concentration camp for most of World War II. While imprisoned, he observed that the people who survived the concentration camps — and only one out of 28 survived — had something they yet wanted to achieve.

After the war, he wrote what the Library of Congress considers one of the 10 most influential books of the 20th century, "Man's Search for Meaning." In it, he argues that man's primary desire is not pleasure, as Sigmund Freud suggested, or power, as Alfred Adler suggested, but meaning and that this, in his darkest hour, is his salvation. He went on to form logotherapy, which is designed to help people discover and pursue their purpose.

Many of you will also be familiar with Stephen Covey's "The 7 Habits of Highly Effective People." He too recognizes the importance of purpose and relationships to successful living. The first three of his habits — start with an end in mind, be proactive and put first things first — all relate to purpose and enable one to move from being dependent to independent. His next three habits — seek first to understand, think win/win and synergize — enable one to move from being independent to interdependent. These three habits all have to do with establishing effective relationships, which is the topic of our next chapter.

(Interestingly, Covey's moving from independence to interdependence is parallel to moving from competition to cooperation or, as Chapter 10 suggests, moving from scarcity to abundance.)

I recognize most all of you have lived with purpose, using your talents to achieve chosen life goals. But how many of us have taken the time to think about those goals, sitting down and writing a page or two about what we wish to accomplish in our lives? Most of us have not looked at our lives in a fully integrated manner, being specific about what we wish to achieve in each of life's domains — family, work, community, and self. The "successful" CEO who has been divorced three times, is estranged from his/her children, is unhealthy, is drinking a little too much and is unhappy didn't set out to achieve this, but rather may have failed to consider what he/she wished to achieve in a fully integrated manner.

I also want to stress that clarifying our purpose is not a one-time endeavor. As life unfolds and progresses, our purpose(s) must evolve too. This is particularly true as we progress through the second half of life. Our work, our family life, our community involvement and we ourselves are all going through major changes requiring us to transition. Successfully navigating these transitions calls for clarity of purpose. If we want to flourish in the second half of life, being clear about what we want to achieve is important. I hope to provide guidance on how to achieve this clarity in the rest of this chapter.

When I work with college students, I tell them, "Purpose is like underwear, don't get caught without it!" In other words, I am challenging them to be sure they are living with a clear purpose. I know from experience that living without purpose does not serve one well. During my first two years of college, I wandered with little direction. When I met my future wife Phyllis the first day of my junior year, I began to realize that I had better start figuring out why I was in college and what I might do after. I began to get clearer about my purpose. My junior and senior years were much more productive and enjoyable.

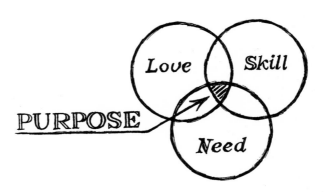

I help students discover their purpose by giving them this quote, modified from Frederick Buechner: "Where your deep gladness, your deep understanding and the world's deep hunger meet." Here's what I think it means: "Your deep gladness" is what you love doing, "your deep understanding" is what you are skilled at, and "the world's deep hunger" is what is needed in the world. Your purpose is at the intersection of what you love doing, what you are skilled at and what the world needs.

In college, I loved to play soccer. The world needs great soccer players. But to tell you the truth, I wasn't very good. The three circles just didn't come together for me. Today, I love the topic of what leads to a flourishing life, I think I am pretty good at sharing my insights about the subject and the world desperately needs more people to flourish. For me, the three circles come together beautifully. My intersection — using my passion and talents to help people flourish — has become a core purpose in my life.

As life unfolds, our purposes can become more challenging, with family, work, community and personal needs often seeming in conflict. The challenge becomes making sure we are thinking about our purpose(s) in an integrated manner so we are not ignoring any aspect of our lives.

Early in my career and well into my 50s, I consistently traded off relationships, specifically with family, for what I thought was my purpose, which revolved too exclusively around work. My guess is many of you do/did the same thing. I think I know why we do this. Many of our objectives at work are tangible and we get measured and rewarded for achieving them. Conversely, relationships are less tangible, with no concrete measures or extrinsic rewards.

Relationships seem to take care of themselves ... until they don't. The challenge as time goes by is how to integrate these seemingly conflicting purposes. People often speak of balancing purpose and relationships. I would rather think in terms of integration. Balance suggests one thing is down, while the other is up. Yes, at times we invariably have to make trade-offs in the short term. But in the longer term, when we integrate the different domains of our lives, we seek to have each domain complement or enhance the other. A key here is defining your purpose in a larger context such that your purpose embraces, or is integrated into, all aspects of your life. When you view your purpose as being one dimensional, you become one dimensional, leading to trade-offs that often come back to haunt you in very painful ways.

When my youngest son Greg was 8 years old, he said one night during dinner, "Dad, we need a suggestion box." I said, "OK." When I came home the next night, there was a suggestion box in the hallway. As we sat down for dinner, Greg said, "Dad, I think there is a suggestion in the suggestion box." I opened the suggestion box and in it was a little yellow sticky note. The message, in Greg's handwriting, read, "I wish Dad had more time to play."

Can you think of a clearer message? "Dad, you ought to spend a little more time at home, and when you are home, you should be present where you are." And still, I traded off relationships for what I thought was my purpose ... work. This yellow sticky note has been on my mirror now for over 30 years.

Or maybe you traded off your personal well-being for work, perhaps not exercising, drinking more than you should, gaining too much weight — basically trading off your health for your wealth. Being clear about what we wish in all of life's domains can help prevent us from making these trade-offs.

As the second half of life unfolds, after the kids leave home and as retirement approaches, our purpose(s) might be challenged by the transitions we experience. Many of us need to find new purposes to replace the ones that governed our days for such a long time.

The three circles presented earlier in this chapter can provide guidance: What do you love doing, what are you skilled at and what does the world need?

Earlier in this book, we spoke about resilience, or how to develop "grit." An important trait of people with grit is that they live with purpose. Having a clear purpose both guides and inspires, helping us move forward with our lives and through any troubles ahead.

Wayne Dyer, known for his books and speeches on self-help and spiritual growth, suggested that "intent" is a force that exists in the universe and that everything has intention, or purpose, built into it. Put another way, every living thing wants to become something — a tadpole, a baby chick, an acorn, the buds on a tree — they are all in harmony with intention, willing participants in this larger whole. We too have the opportunity to tap into this force, but the challenge for us is different. Consider the acorn. It doesn't decide whether or not to have intent. The intent is already completely built into it. Its intent is predetermined. It is programmed to become only one thing … an oak tree. In fact, it can only become a red oak, a white oak, a pin oak — whichever intention is programmed.

We are different. We have intent built into us, but unlike the acorn, our future is not predetermined. We must decide what we are to become. We have the burden of deciding our intent, of choosing to tap into this force, of being clear about what we wish to become, of finding our purpose.

In the second half of life, a key to tapping into the power of intention is moving from ego to conscience, or soul. The ego would have us believe that we are separate from everything else, that we are different from "them," whatever "them" is. Deep within us, however, is an understanding that we are connected to everything else. This understanding leads to kinship, care, love, kindness, bonding. And while all those concepts seem soft, in truth they are amazingly powerful. By moving from ego to soul — by finding purpose(s) with far-reaching benefits to the world and the people around us — we can strengthen our connection to the power of intention. We also become increasingly immune to life's vacillations, the ups and downs, the swirling noise that surrounds us. We become centered, connected, embraced. And that connection to intention can make us a powerful force for good in this world.

For humans, life does not have meaning, rather we give life meaning.

Finding One's Purpose

Answering the abstract question "What is the meaning of life?" will not help you find your purpose. Answering the much more concrete and specific question "What is the meaning of MY life?" will. This is the question each of us must answer if we are to flourish.

To help you find your purpose, I've included at the end of this chapter a three-page worksheet titled "Understanding My Past and Mapping My Future." Let me walk you through filling it out.

1. Begin by reflecting for a few moments about your past. Then try drawing a line that goes from birth to where you are today, considering where you were at different stages in your life. At an age or stage where you felt you were flourishing, your line would be at the top of the chart. At an age or stage that was difficult, your line would be toward the bottom. Identify the events/factors that led to these highs and lows.

2. Next, consider how you responded in the difficult times. Are there strengths that you developed that enabled you to overcome the challenges you faced and

what were the insights you gained or lessons learned? When life seemed great, what types of things were you doing and what talents were you using? Do these times give insight into what you love doing?

3. People who flourish form a resilient or redemptive story about their past — a story that suggests, out of hardship/setbacks comes new growth, new insights, and a deeper more meaningful existence. Write a short redemptive story of your past.

4. Then begin to look forward and consider what you would like to do/be regarding self, family, work and community. Try to write just one sentence about each.

5. Finally, see if you can capture in a sentence what your overall mission is going forward.

You eventually will want to flesh this mission statement out, but this worksheet should provide a good start. You will want to take a "draft mentality" of your mission, as it will evolve over time as life unfolds.

So how do you know if you have found your purpose? I think it is when you begin to wake up in the morning eager to get out of bed, not just because your bladder is calling, but because you are excited to be engaged in something you deeply care about. You feel like what you do utilizes all of your unique talents. In fact, it appears most everything about your past has led to what you are doing. Whatever you are reading, seeing, listening to, the people you interact with, whatever you are experiencing … they all seem connected to what you are engaged in and bring new insights about your purpose. It seems at times like all manner of things come to assist you, such that the synchronicity appears to happen most every day. Finally, what other people think about how you are investing your time and talents seems almost irrelevant as you increasingly listen to your own inner spirit. When you have these feelings, I think you have found and are pursuing your purpose.

My own mission statement follows as a reference. It may stimulate some thoughts for you, but don't spend too much time with it, as each of us has to develop our own unique mission. I try to live my mission statement each day. I never fully make it, but it does guide me and helps me determine how I wish to invest my time and my talents. I am more productive and happier as a result of having this mission.

Douglas A. Smith — Mission

My life, my power, my wisdom, my uniqueness are fulfilled by acting in a manner consistent with this mission.

In a world of scarcity, I will act with abundance. In a world of fear, I will act with love. In a world of anger and retribution, I will act with forgiveness. In a world that is fragmented, I will integrate all aspects of my life. In a world of materialism, I will be guided by my spirit and a concern for what is enduring.

I will grow. I will learn to listen before speaking. I will learn patience. I will increasingly overcome my selfish desires. I will not let the pettiness and the frustration or challenges of the moment mask the significance and the beauty of the gifts and the life I have been given. I will remain appreciative and grateful. I will develop and utilize my talents for the enhancement of this world.

I will serve my family, for it is through them that I create the greatest value. *I will remain faithful to the vows I made to my wife 51 years ago through consistently "loving, honoring, cherishing and serving" her. My wife and I will create a home that is constant and abundant in its love and security, and is therefore conducive to each of us leading successful, meaningful and fulfilling lives. As the primary wage earner, I will provide financial well-being to enable our family to function. Finally, I will remain a friend and support to my extended family and all those with whom I come in contact.*

I will serve my vocation, for it is through work that I develop and direct many of my humble talents. *My work is to understand what leads to a meaningful, flourishing life, to live consistent with this understanding and to help others do the same. First, as a winter term faculty member at DePauw University, I will enhance the lives of the students I serve by sharing my knowledge and experience concerning what it means and how to achieve a flourishing life, such that they can increasingly live considered, consequential and accomplished lives ... to enable them to flourish. Second, as a founder of Positive Foundry, LLC, I will work to bring the science of positive psychology to the corporate world such that organizations we serve and their associates may flourish. I will eventually work to take these same skills to our educational institutions. As an author, I will publish a second book titled "Thriving in the Second Half of Life."*

As a leader of classes at Canyon Ranch and in speaking at various venues across the country, my work here too will be centered on enabling people to thrive. Finally, I will serve as an effective and trusted advisor to various CEOs and leaders of both corporations and not-for-profit organizations, helping these leaders create abundant organizations by clarifying their vision and increasingly engaging their stakeholders in the pursuit of that vision.

I will serve the communities within which I live and work, for it is through this service that I am able to give back a portion of what I have received. *I serve the communities by giving 10% of our income and an increasingly larger percentage of my time to causes that enhance our communities. DePauw University, Dartmouth College, Cristo Rey schools, cancer (particularly blood cancer) and the protection of the Adirondack wilderness are priority areas of my service.*

I will serve the substantive needs of self, for I can only achieve this mission by caring for and nurturing myself. *I do this daily by being physically active, eating well, by nourishing my soul through reflection and worship, and by continuing to expand my mind and vision through continuous learning.*

By fulfilling this mission, I find meaning and value in life, the world finds meaning and value in me, and I find joy in this journey we call life.

Reflections for the Second Half

- Do you feel you can succinctly answer the question "What is the meaning of my life?"

- If the answer is yes, are you living in a manner consistent with that meaning?

Understanding My Past & Mapping My Future

My Life Line

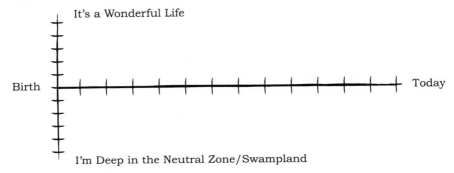

Reflecting Back

Strengths developed:

_____

_____

_____

_____

What I love doing:

_____

_____

_____

_____

Insights gained/lessons learned:

_____

_____

_____

_____

What is the "redemptive story" that emerges from my life?

_____

_____

_____

_____

My Mission

Summary Statement

_____

_____

_____

_____

_____

_____

What do I do for ...

1. Family:

_____

_____

_____

2. Work:

_____

_____

_____

3. Community:

_____

_____

_____

4. Self:

_____

_____

_____

Quotes About Purpose

1. "He who has a reason 'why' to live, can bear most any 'how.'"

—FRIEDRICH NIETZSCHE

2. "This is the one true joy in life, the being used for a purpose recognized by yourself as a mighty one; being a force of nature, instead of a feverish, selfish little clod of ailments and grievances complaining that the world will not devote itself to making you happy."

—GEORGE BERNARD SHAW

3. "To be in hell is to drift; to be in heaven is to steer."

—GEORGE BERNARD SHAW

4. "Life is no brief candle to me. It is a sort of splendid torch which I have got to hold up for the moment, and I want to make it burn as brightly as possible before handing it on to future generations."

—GEORGE BERNARD SHAW

5. "The best moments usually occur when a person's body or mind is stretched to its limits in a voluntary effort to accomplish something difficult and worthwhile. Optimal experience is thus something we make happen."

—MIHALY CSIKSZENTMIHALYI

6. *"Our deepest fear is not that we are inadequate.*
Our deepest fear is that we are powerful beyond
measure.
It is our light, not our darkness
That most frightens us.

…Your playing small
Does not serve the world.
There's nothing enlightened about shrinking
So that other people won't feel insecure around you.

We are all meant to shine,
As children do.
…It's not just in some of us;
It's in everyone.

And as we let our own light shine,
We unconsciously give other people permission to
do the same.
As we're liberated from our own fear,
Our presence automatically liberates others."
                    —MARIANNE WILLIAMSON

7. *"It is not about finding yourself, it is about creat-*
ing yourself."
                    —UNKNOWN

8. *"Make no little plans; they have no magic to stir*
men's blood."
                    —DANIEL BURNHAM

9. *"The place where your deep gladness, [your deep understanding] and the world's hunger meet."*
—FREDERICK BUECHNER
(MODIFIED BY DOUGLAS A. SMITH)

10. *"As a body cannot live without food, so the soul cannot live without purpose."*
—RICHARD ROHR

11. *"The two most important days in your life are the day you are born and the day you find out why."*
—MARK TWAIN

12. *"You can fly, but the cocoon has to go."*
—ANONYMOUS

13. *"The moment one definitely commits oneself, then Providence moves too. All sorts of things occur to help one that would never otherwise have occurred. A whole stream of events issues from the decision, raising in one's favor all manner of unforeseen incidents and meetings and material assistance, which no man could have dreamed would have come his way. Whatever you do, or dream you can, begin it. Boldness has genius, power, and magic in it. "*
—GOETHE

Chapter 13

CHERISHING RELATIONSHIPS

A life is not important except in the impact it has on other lives.

—JACKIE ROBINSON'S TOMBSTONE

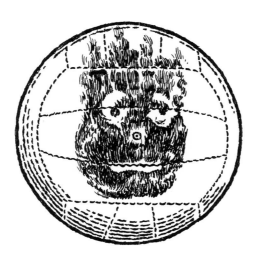

Let's go back to the movie "Cast Away" and the second prop identified: the soccer ball.

One of the packages that washes up on the beach of the deserted island contains a soccer ball. Unsure what to do with it, Chuck Noland puts it aside. Several days later, after he has left a bloody handprint on the ball, he makes it into a face and begins to call the ball "Wilson." Wilson from then on is a constant companion. When he leaves the island, he takes Wilson with him on a makeshift raft. After several weeks on the raft, he wakes to find Wilson drifting away. He swims after Wilson while holding a vine fashioned into a rope. Wilson is drifting one way and the raft the other. He can't quite get to Wilson and must decide to either let go of the "rope" and go with Wilson, in which case he will drown, or go back to the raft. He is torn and eventually swims back to the raft, but at this point he is devastated and basically gives up hope. Wilson, of course, represents the importance of relationships.

Relationships have been key to survival throughout human history. We often talk about survival of the fittest, but when you think about it, we are not a very impressive physical species. We don't have sharp claws or teeth, we aren't particularly strong, and we can't run as fast as most of our predators. In prehistoric times, alone we made a pretty good target or meal. It is collectively that we were powerful. What enabled humans to survive 100,000 years ago was the ability to come together, to cooperate, to be in a relationship, to care for and about one another ... to love. Bound together, we suddenly had the strength to protect ourselves and become the hunter rather than the hunted. At our core, we are wired to be in relation to others. The better our relationships, the more likely we are to flourish.

At the core of better relationships is the skill of emotional intelligence. Most of us have heard the term and have a general idea of what it means, but most of us are not familiar with the competencies and skills that comprise this wonderful capability. Let me cover emotional intelligence in a little more detail.

Emotional intelligence (EQ) determines, to a large degree, how well we relate to and interact with others. Unlike IQ, our EQ can be enhanced. For most of us, it improves as we age. And, like any skill, we can also study it, better understand what it is and learn new ways to enhance it, and thereby enhance our relationships. Since having enduring relationships is a primary factor in enabling us to flourish, EQ then plays an important role in flourishing.

Having a high EQ requires both personal competence and social competence. Personal competence, or how effectively we deal with ourselves, requires the skills of self-awareness and self-management. Social competence, or how effectively we deal with others, requires the skills of social awareness and relationship management.

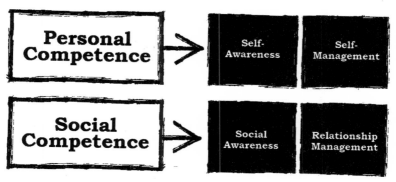

Source: "Emotional Intelligence Quick Book," Travis Bradberry and Jean Greaves

Self-awareness is accurately understanding how we feel and, specifically, why we feel this way. A person with a high degree of self-awareness will not just recognize that they are feeling upset or feeling badly, they will know whether they are feeling nervous, overwhelmed, undervalued, pressured, anxious, incompetent, etc. They understand their emotions at a deep enough level that they can then begin to pinpoint why they feel this way. A person with high self-awareness might surmise, "I often feel pressured when I have a deadline to meet" or "I often feel incompetent when I am talking about statistics and analytical problems." This type of self-awareness requires that we know ourselves well and that we have the self-confidence, or self-esteem, that permits us to recognize and accept feelings that may well be negative, or that we view as undesirable.

Self-management determines how we act (or don't act) as a result of our feelings. It is the ability to act in a manner that is constructive. Many of us when we feel anger will strike out, expressing our anger aggressively, or we completely withdraw from discussion without spending the time to consider if there are more positive and productive ways to handle our emotions. Self-management is the ability to constructively steer our responses to people and situations in ways that work to our advantage. When we express anger in an appropriate and constructive manner it serves to channel our energy toward resolving issues rather than into attacking another person. Self-management is also the ability to avoid situations that put us in a negative position. For instance, if we know we will feel pressured when there's a deadline to meet, we would work to do things well in advance to minimize the pressure of the deadline.

Social competence focuses on our ability to understand others and to manage relationships. The first skill is **social awareness**. It is having the empathy to understand what others are thinking and feeling. It is the ability to see beyond our own emotions and consider the emotions of others. **Relationship management** is the ability to use that knowledge of what others are feeling to make relationships more effective. A person with excellent relationship management skills will connect with others, even those that they may not agree with or those they are not particularly fond of. They find ways to effectively relate to and engage with others.

A first step, in emotional intelligence is managing your emotions to not be of harm to yourself or others. A second, more difficult step is learning to manage your emotions to benefit yourself and everyone with whom you come in contact.

According to Daniel Goleman, author of "Emotional Intelligence: Why It Can Matter More Than IQ," people with high EQs exhibit these qualities: self-confidence, self-esteem, trustworthiness, empathy, patience, caring, persuasiveness, leadership and the ability to work in teams. Seems like a pretty good list!

Source: "What Makes a Leader?" Daniel Goleman, Harvard Business Review, June 1996

How to Practice Effective Relationships

Here are several tools that can help you build better relationships:

1. Improve your EQ. This was covered in some detail in this chapter, and these books may also be helpful:

"Emotional Intelligence Quick Book" by Travis Bradberry and Jean Greaves, "Emotional Intelligence 2.0" by Travis Bradberry and Jean Greaves, and "Emotional Intelligence: Why It Can Matter More Than IQ" by Daniel Goleman.

2. Devote all 140 bits of information capability to the other person. This is a simple tool to help you listen better. Hearing and listening are not the same. Hearing is the recognition of a sound. Listening requires that we make an effort to understand what the sound means. To listen we must focus, take time and care to understand the emotions and the intent behind the words expressed. Psychologists have suggested that our minds are capable of handling about 140 bits of information per second. Casual conversation takes about 40. And what do most of us do while in conversation? If you are like me, you begin to use the remaining 100 bits of information to think about tomorrow, what happened yesterday, maybe check your phone for messages, daydream, etc. But if you devote all 140 bits of your capability to one other person — a spouse, a son or daughter, a co-worker, your boss — and give them your total attention, you will make a friend for life. Why? Because no one does it. It is hard to do, but try it. Give someone all 140 bits of information capability. You will be amazed at the response.

3. Increase your "Emotional Bank Account." Every time you interact with another person in a positive way, you are making a deposit in what Stephen Covey calls your "emotional bank account" with that person. When we have a negative interaction — break a commitment, strike out in anger inappropriately, gossip about them — we make a withdrawal from that emotional bank account. Over time this is the way relationships are built or destroyed. If you raise what is known as your "Jen Ratio," you will improve your relationships. The Jen Ratio is simply the measure of positive interactions to negative interactions. One can measure this between two people, within a team, at home, at work, at school, etc. Psychologists have determined the different ratios required in different settings.

For instance, at work, the Jen Ratio is referred to as the "Losada Ratio" and the magic ratio is 3:1. Companies that flourish have a ratio of at least 3:1, but not higher than 12:1. If the ratio is above 12:1 — that's more than 12 positive interactions to one negative interaction — the organization is not facing reality or having the conflict necessary for success. In a marriage, the Jen Ratio is called the "Gottman Ratio." For marriages to flourish, the ratio needs to be at least 5:1. For friends, it needs to be 3:1. To build better relationships, you need to maximize your deposits and minimize the withdrawals.

4. Practice "Active Constructive Responding." There are four potential ways you can respond to someone when they share good news with you. Only one of the four — active constructive responding — leads to better relationships, and many of us fail to practice it. Below is a chart that shows the four ways to respond and an example of each response.

	CONSTRUCTIVE	DESTRUCTIVE
ACTIVE	"Let Them Savor"	"Ruin Their Experience"
PASSIVE	"Gently Deflate Them" [Who Cares]	"It's ALL About Me"

Source: Researcher Shelly Gable and colleagues

Here is an example of each type of response when someone tells you they are going to Mexico on vacation:

	CONSTRUCTIVE	DESTRUCTIVE
ACTIVE	"That's great — tell me more!"	"Isn't there a problem with crime?"
PASSIVE	"Oh, cool."	"I am going to the Bahamas!"

From my own experience, it is so easy to fall into any of the three quadrants that are not "active constructive responding." Put simply, when someone shares good news with you, the only appropriate response is, "Tell me more!"

5. "Companioning." When someone tells me they are having a difficult time, my natural response is to jump in and try to help them figure out how to deal with their challenges. That's not always a good idea. I'd be better off "companioning." Companioning is a concept outlined in Sheryl Sandberg's excellent book "Option B: Facing Adversity, Building Resilience and Finding Joy." When someone else is struggling, our first response should simply be being there for them, being present and showing empathy. Sandberg's point is that when someone is struggling, they may not yet be ready to begin searching for solutions, they may just be coming to accept the situation. At that point, just being a companion, letting the person know that we care and are prepared to be there for them as a companion is a more helpful strategy. When we are challenged it helps to know that we are not alone, that we have a companion.

6. Risk being vulnerable. To have effective relationships, you must be willing to be vulnerable. Effective relationships are built on trust. You trust someone when you know you can share with them information that they could use to hurt you and they don't do so. In other words, when you make yourself vulnerable and they, in turn, handle that information in a caring manner. Trust requires some level of vulnerability. When we communicate at a meaningful level, we form deeper more enduring relationships. When you are willing to answer some of the personal questions below, you are making yourself vulnerable:

• What is your greatest fear?

- What matters to you the most?

- What are your greatest strengths? Your biggest weaknesses?

- What is the most powerful emotion you have felt in the past year? What were the circumstances?

7. Let go of the negative. Most of us cherish and keep close our little grudges like we would our favorite pets. When we continuously complain, we actually start noticing more things to complain about. Our negative thoughts rewire our brain to seek out the worst, and that discourages others from being close to us.

8. Have more "I-Thou" relationships. In most encounters with others, our minds tend to objectify the other person. That is, we often view others as a vehicle to achieve something. Philosopher Martin Buber called this an "I-It" relationship. An I-It relationship is probably appropriate when we call a 1-800 number to order a sweatshirt. But too often we treat relationships as I-It when they deserve to be much broader and deeper. We should strive to have more of what Buber calls "I-Thou" relationships, where we don't view our interaction with others as transactional. An I-Thou relationship is ripe with opportunity to understand the other person in their full complexity and seeks pathways, not only to their minds, but also to their hearts and souls. I-Thou relationships open our minds, hearts and souls and lead to better relationships and greater joy.

9. Put the phone down! In fact, put it out of sight and out of earshot. The average teenager sends more than 3,100 text messages a month. That is more than

100 a day. Many of us may send about the same number. Why? Why do we choose to text the person across the table rather than speak with them? Could it be because a social media friend provides "faux intimacy," a relationship where we don't really need to engage with them, share who we really are, what we care about, what we love or fear, or what we believe and hold dear? With texting, we can stay in the shallows and not risk hurting someone else or getting hurt in the process. We get a nice dopamine boost without being vulnerable. But social media relationships offer little enduring gratification and leave us feeling alone. Put the phone down and take the risk of developing deeper relationships, relationships that enable us to flourish even in times of crisis.

10. Ask back. When someone asks you a question — "Where did you go to school?" or "Where did you grow up?" or "What type of work do you do?" — they are curious, but they often have something they would like to share about the same topic. Ask them the same question. I often get so wrapped up in my answer to their question, I fail to ask back and miss an opportunity to form a closer relationship.

11. Be assertive. In our relationships with others, we need to be assertive, not passive or aggressive. When we are passive, we don't honor our own feelings, thoughts and needs. When we are aggressive, we don't honor the feelings, thoughts and needs of others. When we are assertive, we respect ourselves and others.

12. RASA: This is a concept from Julian Treasure, author of "How to Be Heard." "Rasa" is a Sanskrit word meaning essence. Treasure used the acronym RASA as a tool for listening. Treasure suggests when someone speaks we should first **Receive** whatever they are saying with as few filters as possible; then **Appreciate** what they are saying with verbal cues to them like "un-huh," "yes," "I understand;" then **Summarize** in our own words what they are saying; and then **Ask** questions for clarity.

13. Practice the 13 skills covered in this book. Each of the 13 skills leads to better relationships.

Reflections for the Second Half

- Do the relationships with those closest to you bring you joy? Would you like to improve some of these relationships?

- Do you see how you could have even better relationships by developing and practicing the skills covered in this chapter?

Quotes About Relationships

1. "A life is not important except in the impact it has on other lives."

—JACKIE ROBINSON'S TOMBSTONE

2. "The most important factor in the survival of Homo sapiens is our social nature, our ability to love one another and work together."

—ELLEN BERSCHEID

3. "Numerous studies show that intimate relationships, such as marriages, are the single most important source of life satisfaction."

—SUZANN PILEGGI

4. "Psychologists agree that IQ contributes only about 20% of the factors that determine success. A full 80% comes from other factors, including what I call emotional intelligence."

—DANIEL GOLEMAN,
"EMOTIONAL INTELLIGENCE"

5. "You cannot paint sunlight; you can only capture the effect it has on other objects."

—WILLA CATHER

6. *"The effect of the injury appears to have been the destruction of the equilibrium between his intellectual faculties and the animal propensities. He was now capricious, fitful, irreverent, impatient of restraint, vacillating ... The balance of his mind was gone."*
—DR. JOHN MARTYN HARLOW WRITING ABOUT PHINEAS GAGE

7. *"Some cause happiness wherever they go, others, whenever they go."*
—OSCAR WILDE

8. *"We are a 'face-to-face' species. We are a 'caretaking' species. Our hierarchies differ from other species. Power goes to the most emotionally intelligent. We reconcile conflicts rather than fleeing or killing. We have evolved powerful capacities to forgive."*
—DACHER KELTNER

9. *"Happiness to a raindrop is joining the river."*
—UNKNOWN

Chapter 14

DEAD ENDS

The essential trick of the happiness traps is that they seem to offer the solution to happiness, even as they destroy any chance of ever achieving it. One of the cruelest paradoxes of life is that the things we so often seek to soothe our souls are the very things that ultimately feed our fears and cause happiness to forever recede before us, just out of reach.
—DAN BAKER, "WHAT HAPPY PEOPLE KNOW"

Dead ends are pathways we choose that lead us nowhere. My guess is you will recognize most of them because you probably have traveled down them at one time or another. We may experience them and then recalibrate our lives to avoid them. But to the degree we continue to travel down dead ends, they take an increasing toll on our ability to flourish. The more we succumb to dead ends, the more damage accumulates, affecting us and those around us. Avoiding dead ends is a key to flourishing. Often dead ends look like shortcuts to happiness, but they usually lead instead to downright misery. Dead ends are easy to recognize, but very hard to get out of. I know because I have traveled down each of them.

Here are five common dead ends that can divert you from the path to a flourishing life:

1. The "Pleasure" Dead End

This dead end ensnares most of us and often leads to misery. We hurt ourselves, and those we love, when pleasure is pursued too aggressively or compulsively. Seneca had it right: "Pleasure is the happiness of a madman."

In the second half of life we are particularly vulnerable to this dead end. After our children leave home and/or our professional responsibilities diminish, we often turn to alcohol to fill the void. Binge drinking among college students is a problem, but the highest rate of binge drinking is among those aged 65 and over.

Pleasure does not equal happiness. It is a factor of both happiness and a flourishing life, but only a factor. In fact, pleasure is the dessert of happiness and a flourishing life, not the main course. Yes, it is a part of happiness, but it can never be the foundation because it has some peculiar traits that make it hard — if not impossible — to bring us any lasting sense of well-being. Because of these traits, when we make pleasure too large a part of our lives, some strange and unpleasant things begin to happen.

Here is what we know about pleasure:

- It feels good.

- It can be the result of stimulus added or taken away, but it depends on an external stimulus.

- Bodily pleasure centers on the access points to our bodies.

And here is where the trouble begins:

- Pleasure can be chemically replicated.

- It is the change in stimulus that gives pleasure.

- We adapt to it through a process known as "habituation," or "adaptation." Once we are used to the pleasure, it no longer has the capability to make us happy until there is a further change in stimulus.

Neither the drug addict nor the alcoholic is happy. Both are bound up in the relentless pursuit of a feeling that seems just beyond their reach. When pleasure becomes the meal, rather than the dessert, it's a problem. Addicts don't take drugs to feel high, they take drugs in an attempt to not feel bad.

2. The "Money/Prestige/Success/Praise" Dead End

Why is it so hard for all of us (including me) to accept that money doesn't buy happiness? Probably because, to some extent, money does buy happiness. Poverty is not fun. As many people have said, "I have been rich and I have been poor ... rich is better." In fact, happiness and annual income levels do increase rather nicely together up to a household income of $60,000 to $70,000. From there, the correlation begins to weaken, and after about $150,000 there is almost no correlation.

If that statistic doesn't stop us from thinking more money will bring more happiness, here's another that might: Since 1950 the U.S. GNP (gross national product) per capita in constant dollars has gone up threefold. Meanwhile, the percentage of people who say they are very or somewhat happy has marginally decreased and the percentage of people who will experience a major depression during their lifetimes has gone up tenfold. One of the most pervasive and persuasive myths in our society is that "more will make us happier." Too few recognize this is a myth. The causative link between money and happiness, particularly for those at the upper income levels, is spurious, but oh how firmly we believe it.

It is hard to buy happiness with money partly because of a survival instinct known as "psychological homeostasis," which is our tendency to quickly adjust to life circumstances, both bad and good. So the happiness we feel when we first buy a new car quickly fades and we return to feeling the way we did before.

Don't get me wrong, I am not suggesting that money and what we do with it is not important. The responsible use of money is critical to happiness. When I talk with my college students, I suggest that money is an important resource in life. They should earn it, save a portion and invest it wisely. I also tell them they should take out a loan for only three reasons: to buy a house, to get an education and to buy a car, if they can't get to work without one. They should have no other loans and under NO circumstances should they have debt on their credit cards. But if we are waiting for more money to bring us happiness, it won't happen. Think of it this way: The happy rich person was happy before they were rich.

Like money, prestige, status, professional success and

the praise of others can also be sought out as routes to happiness. We tend to think happiness will come from gaining prestige over others, often through the accumulation of material goods or through promotions, titles or social recognition. Unfortunately, the desire to accumulate goods and climb the social ladder are an instinctive part of our biological makeup. In our former hunter-gatherer society, which accounts for about 90% of the time humans have been on the planet, some individuals dominated because they were better at getting and keeping scarce resources.

However, people in so-called "low status" occupations are about as happy as those in "high status" positions. Again, I am not suggesting that the prestige, promotions and financial rewards earned through success at work are not to be enjoyed. They should be. But to flourish we also need forgiveness, gratitude, altruism/kindness, healthy relationships ... we need to practice the 13 skills covered in this book. Money by itself doesn't buy happiness.

There is one specific way that money can buy enduring happiness ... when we use it for the benefit of others. I am sure Bill Gates and Warren Buffett get a meaningful boost in their happiness through the use of their resources to benefit people across the world through the Bill & Melinda Gates Foundation. Altruism is a sure path to happiness.

3. The "Sympathy" Dead End

Strange as it seems, many of us tend to seek happiness in sympathy. We look for others to raise us up by expressing how terrible our plight is. This dead end is attractive because we become the center of attention and we relieve ourselves of the responsibility to do something about our predicament as others affirm we are in a bad place.

With setbacks in life it is normal, in fact necessary, to grieve. But when we hang on to grief or sorrow for an extended period, it becomes a blanket for us to hide under. By moving to Pity City we make ourselves victims, and victims are not happy or flourishing individuals. Remember, we have the ability to master our own stories and decide whether or not to be a victim. Ask yourself, "What is the story of my life? Is it the story of a victim or one of redemption and resilience?"

Sorrow is a natural stage when we experience a setback. But it cannot become a destination if we want to flourish. It is okay to visit Pity City, you just can't move there.

4. The "Now" Dead End

This dead end occurs when we make decisions that lead to feeling good now, but cause a lot of pain later. For instance, think of the purchase that is instantly gratifying but stretches far beyond your means.

Few among us consciously ask ourselves, "Will this decision/action make me happier or enable me to flourish in the long run?" Instead, we often dive into whatever it is that would seem to fulfill the desires of the moment ... what we want NOW ... and in so doing we end up trading off something that is considerably more important to us in the longer term. Most of us play the "should/shouldn't game" — I should do this, but don't; I shouldn't do this, but do.

In the 1960s, Walter Mischel conducted a well-known study with 4-year-old kids in which he put each in a room with a marshmallow. He said he would be stepping out of the room and returning in 15 minutes, and if they could refrain from eating the marshmallow during that time, he would give them a second marshmallow when he returned. He also gave some of the kids strategies to succeed. He then followed the kids for the next 14 years. Those that best used the strategies and could wait — those that didn't fall into the "now" dead end — experienced more success academically and socially in later years.

This doesn't mean we should never go to the party that keeps us from studying or that we should never have dessert, but we should be conscious of the trade-offs we are making when we make decisions. We should never trade what we want most (to graduate/to stay healthy) for what we want now (to party/to eat dessert).

5. The "When/If" Dead End

Many of us put a "when" or an "if " around happiness. I will be happy WHEN I get the next promotion ... when I finish this assignment ... when I leave for vacation ... when the kids leave for college. Or I would be happy IF my husband would treat me better ... if I get the big promotion/pay raise ... if I could lose 30 pounds ... if I could have a child. By putting a "when" or an "if" before our happiness, we are putting off happiness into some distant future, or worse, putting our happiness into someone else's hands.

Here is the stark reality: No one and nothing is coming to make us happy. Happiness is an inside job. We create our own happiness. Possessions, titles, raises, accolades, money, vacations, houses, cars will bring a momentary feeling of happiness, but they do not sustain us. Enduring, authentic happiness is a perspective, an attitude that we create for ourselves; it is not dependent on someone or something else. Still, most of us have a "wait problem," putting off our happiness for some future time or event.

Happiness is not in the future and it is not outside of us. Happiness is in the present and inside of us.

Reflections for the Second Half

- Which of the dead ends do you feel you are most vulnerable to?

- Can you give examples of when you stepped into one of these dead ends? How did it feel?

- Why are these dead ends so hard to avoid?

- What actions might you take in the future to avoid heading down these dead ends?

Quotes About Dead Ends

1. *"Every pleasure carries with it the seeds of its own destruction."*

—ARISTOTLE

2. *"Happy successful people were happy before they were successful."*

—DOUGLAS A. SMITH

3. *"The main cause of failure and unhappiness is trading what we want most for what we want now."*

—ZIG ZIGLAR

4. *"Pleasure is the happiness of madmen, while happiness is the pleasure of sages."*

—JULES BARBEY D'AUREVILLY

5. *"How strange would appear to be this thing that men call pleasure. And how curiously it is related to what is thought to be its opposite, pain. Wherever the one is found, the other follows up behind."*

—PLATO

6. *"Don't tell your problems to people; 80% don't care ... and the other 20% are glad you have them."*

—LOU HOLTZ

7. *"All we really ever want is everything."*
—DOUGLAS A. SMITH

8. *"There are things that I can't leave alone, Cause they won't leave me alone. Cause what I want ain't what I need, Still I reach for things I crave. Better try to run away, Am I afraid of being free? You tell me. Cause when I'm not chasing demons, There's demons chasing me."*
—KENNY CHESNEY, "DEMONS"

9. *"It is generally good for your happiness to have money, but toxic to your happiness to want money too much."*
—ED DIENER

10. *"Success is not the key to happiness. Happiness is the key to success."*
—ALBERT SCHWEITZER

11. *"Money can't buy you happiness. But happiness just might buy you money."*
—DOUGLAS A. SMITH

Chapter 15

LOVE

Love. This is the wellspring of happiness, renewable and everlasting. Love is the polar opposite of fear, emotionally and neurologically. Thus, it is the antidote to fear and the first step toward happiness.

—DAN BAKER

So far, we've talked about 13 skills that, when practiced and mastered, can lead to thriving in the second half of life. All of them — from forgiveness, to gratitude, to altruism, to abundance — are fueled by one common denominator: love. Without love, our search for happiness and our desire to flourish are in vain. Love is the 14th skill.

When we live in a world of anger, win/ lose competition, entitlement, judgment, scarcity — a world driven by fear — it is difficult, if not impossible, to flourish. I know this because for most of my life I was often driven by fear. My fears included failing to get into my chosen college, not getting a desired job or promotion, being afraid of getting fired, not being able to provide for my family, not being successful enough in other people's eyes, etc. You are probably familiar with these fears. They drove me to study hard, to work hard, and to accumulate wealth. They drove me to be successful by many common measures. However, it is hard, if not impossible, to flourish, to be happy, if you are driven by fear.

Dan Baker, in his book "What Happy People Know," identified two powerful fears that drive most of us: "I won't BE enough" and "I won't HAVE enough." Ironically, when we are driven by these fears, we will never be enough or have enough. We will be haunted by these fears even as we fly in our private Lear jet to our fourth multimillion-dollar home. We will always feel as if the price of our security is our insecurity ... which means we will never be secure.

We don't have to give up our edge or our ability to be successful by giving up these fears. In fact, I think to the degree we give up these fears and are inspired by love, we will be even more successful. Why? Because so few people are inspired by love. Being inspired by love will make you unique in a fragmented, scarcity, fear-driven world. If love is at the center of your life and you emanate care and concern for those around you, it becomes a virtuous circle. Love will flow back to you. Others will want to help and support you, to assist you in whatever you pursue.

I think with each moment we are challenged to make a choice between being inspired by love or driven by fear. No one can make these choices for us. While this may seem daunting, the next moment also provides us a new opportunity to make a better choice.

Below is a chart with each of the 13 skills based on love and its counterpoint based in fear. Flourishing, I believe, is living on the left side by putting love at the center of our lives and letting love guide our decisions and actions.

CHOOSING LOVE

LOVE	FEAR
Forgiveness	Anger/Vengeance
Gratitude	Entitlement
Faith	Doubt
Optimism	Pessimism
Flexibility	Rigidity
Openness	Denial
Doing Now What I Am Doing	Multi-tasking
Honoring Mind/Body/Spirit	Disregarding Mind/Body/Spirit
Altruism/Kindness	Bitterness/Selfishness
Abundance/Cooperation	Scarcity/Competition
Mastering Our Stories	Slave to Our Inner Voice
Finding Meaning/Purpose	Drifting
Cherishing Relationships	Dysfunctional Relationships

If we live with love, we will care for ourselves, care for others and care for the world we all inhabit. When we put love at the center of our lives, we will accept others as they are; we will forgive ourselves and others; we will prepare for the future, while accepting that we cannot control the future; we will be kind; we will live with gratitude; we will think with abundance; we will use our talents to help others; we will live with purpose and cherish our relationships; ... we will have peace with our past, confidence in our future and live with joy in the present. We will thrive.

As I write this in the early months of 2020 and I am sheltered in place at home because of the COVID-19 pandemic, it clearly dawns on me how grateful I am for just being alive and with family. Last night I watched "Everyone Loves Raymond." My oldest son Gordon loves the show and almost every night we watch a couple of episodes together. I think I've seen each episode at least four or five times. It is not that I love the show that much, it is that I love my son Gordon that much. It is a joy to watch him laugh as the show unfolds and to hear his comments about what is happening.

This morning we received from my youngest son Greg and his wife Nicole a short video of their daughter, our 3-year-old grandchild Elaine, singing "Humpty Dumpty," with gentle coaching from Greg, while she randomly stroked the strings of a guitar. My wife, Gordon and I laughed and were filled with delight. As I watched the video and Phyllis's reaction, I realized how blessed I am that Greg and Nicole are such incredible parents, and that I have shared a marriage with Phyllis for 51 years. These simple pleasures are ones I would have failed to fully appreciate in the first half of life.

May you choose to be inspired by love and may you thrive in the second half of your life.

Reflections for the Second Half

- Reflecting back on your own life, were your actions driven by fear or inspired by love?

- Looking forward, are there ways you can move even closer to being inspired by love?

Quotes About Love

1. "Relationships are the key to happiness. Happiness is love. Full Stop."

—GEORGE VAILLANT

2. "A thought transfixed me: for the first time in my life I saw the truth as it is set into song by so many poets, proclaimed as the final wisdom by so many thinkers. The truth — that love is the ultimate and highest goal to which man can aspire. I grasped the meaning of the greatest secret that human poetry and human thought and belief have to impart. The salvation of man is through love and in love."

—VIKTOR FRANKL

3. "Above all else, flourishing is a love of life and a life of love."

—DOUGLAS A. SMITH

4. "When all your desires are distilled, you will cast just two votes: To love more and be happy."

—HAFIZ

5. "The essence of all religions is love, tolerance and compassion. Kindness is my true religion."

—DALAI LAMA

6. *"Fear is the cheapest room in the house. I would like to see you living in better conditions."*

—HAFIZ

7. *"We are not a particularly impressive physical animal. We do not have the benefit of natural weaponry, armor, strength, flight, stealth, or speed relative to many other species. It is our ability to reason, plan and work together that sets us apart from other animals. Human survival depends on our collective abilities, our ability to join together with others in pursuing a goal, not on our individual might."*

—JOHN CACIOPPO [FROM "FLOURISH" BY MARTIN SELIGMAN, PAGE 145]

8. *"Human goodness [love] may be stronger than any other instinct or motive."*

—CHARLES DARWIN

9. *"Survival of the kindest may be just as fitting a description of our origins as survival of the fittest."*

—DACHER KELTNER

10. *"Love. This is the wellspring of happiness, renewable and everlasting. Love is the polar opposite of fear, emotionally and neurologically. Thus, it is the antidote to fear and the first step toward happiness."*

—DAN BAKER

11. "So I say to you, walk with the wind, brothers and sisters, and let the spirit of peace and the power of everlasting love be your guide."

—JOHN LEWIS

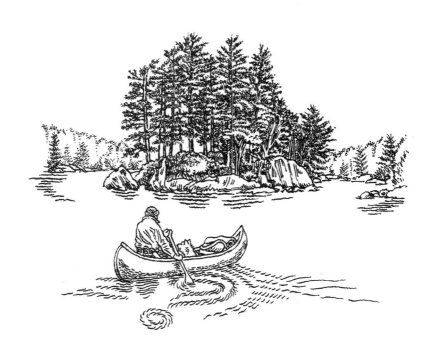

APPENDIX

Appendix

MEET THE AUTHORS

BEHIND THE WORDS

Choose an author as you would a friend.

—Wentworth Dillon

Douglas A. Smith

Doug, a former business leader, is relishing the second half of his life as a speaker, teacher, writer and business co-founder. In his previous life, he served as CEO of Kraft Foods Canada, Chairman/CEO of Borden Foods Corporation and Chairman/CEO of Best Brands Corporation.

His specific areas of interest are leadership and organizational effectiveness, happiness and well-being, and the skill of dealing with setbacks in life. He works with organizations and individuals, focusing on emerging companies, as well as CEOs who are eager to learn and enhance their leadership skills and live with greater joy and abundance.

Doug's interest in positive psychology led him to author a best-selling book titled "Happiness: The Art of Living with Peace, Confidence and Joy" (released January 2014). He teaches an undergraduate course at DePauw University and leads sessions at Canyon Ranch on "The Science & Skill of Happiness" and "Thriving in the Second Half of Life." Doug speaks on both leadership and happiness at conferences and organizations across the country and consults with numerous CEOs. He is also a popular speaker at business meetings and conventions. He donates 100% of his fees and 100% of his book profits to charitable organizations involved in cancer research, the environment or education. To date, his work and writing have raised over $1.5 million for these causes. Most recently, he co-founded Positive Foundry, an organization dedicated to enabling individuals and their organizations to flourish.

Doug has a BA and an honorary doctorate from DePauw University and an MBA from Dartmouth College. Doug and his wife Phyllis live in Columbus, Ohio, and have two grown sons, a wonderful daughter-in-law and an adorable granddaughter. Should you wish to reach him, you can find him at whitepinemountain.com.

Kenneth F. Murphy

Ken, a former senior executive, has shifted gears in the second half of life to pursue creativity in writing, photography and filmmaking — all in the service of telling stories of dramatic challenge and growth. He previously served as Senior VP of Human Resources for the Altria Group of companies and in the top human resources role for Kraft Foods Canada with Doug.

In his corporate life, Ken was as a professional coach and advisor to more than 30 senior-level executives. As a teacher within his firms, he developed and successfully integrated the use of the arts into corporate leadership initiatives, with a focus on theater, film, history, and philosophy. This lifelong focus on the liberal arts led to a major shift when he turned 50.

Wishing to tell stories himself rather than simply build off the creative efforts of others, Ken pursued an MFA degree from Columbia University's School of the Arts in the film division.

Ken's feature-length screenplay "Fire on the Beach" was awarded Faculty Honors at the 2012 Columbia

University Film Festival, one of only 11 scripts selected for that distinction. He produced the award-winning short film "First Match," for which he received the 2010 HBO Young Producer's Development Award. The film premiered at the 2011 New York Film Festival at Lincoln Center. Ken wrote and directed the award-winning short film "Reaching Home," featuring Broadway, film and television veteran Debra Monk. Most recently, he has completed his third feature-length screenplay, also entitled "Reaching Home."

In addition to his work at Columbia, Ken has a BS in Industrial & Labor Relations from Cornell University. He and his wife Ginny have enjoyed living in Fairfield, Connecticut, for more than 35 years.